PRINCIPLES OF DRUG DISPOSITION IN DOMESTIC ANIMALS:

The Basis of Veterinary Clinical Pharmacology

J. DESMOND BAGGOT, B.Sc., M.V.B., M.V.M., Ph.D., M.R.C.V.S.

School of Veterinary Studies
Murdoch University
Western Australia

Formerly Associate Professor of Pharmacology
and Veterinary Clinical Sciences
The Ohio State University
Columbus, Ohio

1977   W. B. SAUNDERS COMPANY
Philadelphia • London • Toronto

W. B. Saunders Company: West Washington Square
Philadelphia, Pa. 19105

1 St. Anne's Road
Eastbourne, East Sussex BN21 3UN, England

1 Goldthorne Avenue
Toronto, Ontario M8Z 5T9, Canada

Library of Congress Cataloging in Publication Data

Baggot, J   Desmond.

Principles of drug disposition in domestic animals.

1. Veterinary pharmacology.   I. Title.   [DNLM:
1. Drug therapy—Veterinary.   2. Pharmacology.
3. Animals, Domestic.   SF915 B144p]

SF915.B25   636.089'5   76–54036

ISBN 0–7216–1473–6

Principles of Drug Disposition in Domestic Animals   ISBN   0-7216-1473-6

© 1977 by W. B. Saunders Company.   Copyright under the International Copyright
Union.   All rights reserved.   This book is protected by copyright.   No part of it may
be reproduced, stored in a retrieval system, or transmitted in any form or by any means,
electronic, mechanical, photocopying, recording, or otherwise, without written per-
mission from the publisher.   Made in the United States of America.   Press of W. B.
Saunders Company.   Library of Congress Catalog card number 76-54036.

Last digit is the print number: 9   8   7   6   5   4   3   2   1

Preface

Clinical pharmacology is now widely accepted as an important discipline in medical science. It is a broadly based discipline in that it presumes knowledge of the structures and functions of the systems of the body, explains alteration of chemical compounds by enzyme activity, and binding of drug molecules to tissue constituents in biochemical terms, and it applies the concepts of pharmacokinetics. Differential calculus is the language of pharmacokinetics, which attempts to describe the time course of drug (and metabolite) levels in the fluids, tissues, and excreta of the body. An understanding of the influence of disease states (uremia, fever) and particular conditions (congestive heart failure, diabetes mellitus) on the distribution, fate and clearance of therapeutic agents is presently being sought.

Despite the widespread use of drugs in domestic animals (e.g., in livestock production, as therapeutic and anesthetic agents, in research and the development of drug products), most schools of veterinary medicine put little emphasis on clinical pharmacology in their curricula. In addition to individual variations in organ function and enzyme activity, there are distinct anatomical and physiological differences among the species of domestic animals. Species differences in response to drugs can usually be attributed to differences in their absorption, distribution, biotransformation and excretion, but may sometimes be due to inherent differences in tissue sensitivity. The diversity of animal species makes veterinary clinical pharmacology a most interesting, though rather complex, discipline.

A crucial question in any clinical situation is whether or not to administer a drug. If the answer is affirmative, dosage with the appropriate drug product should be based on relevant pharmacokinetic data.

It is my belief that dosage required to give optimum effectiveness can either be derived mathematically or be determined from several years of clinical evaluation. Both methods, however, require actual experience, since in the former method a therapeutic range of levels (or at least that which gives maximum and safe effect) must be defined. When drugs are given irrationally (including unnecessarily) or used in such a manner that they constitute an environmental hazard, it reflects on the scientific background of the individual who administers them or recommends their use.

I wish to acknowledge the enormous contribution made by Lloyd E. Davis, D.V.M., Ph.D., to comparative pharmacology, and his unceasing efforts to increase awareness by agricultural, medical and veterinary scientists of the significance of clinical pharmacology in veterinary medicine. The support and encouragement which Lloyd has given me since 1969 are deeply appreciated.

This book was prepared under rather difficult circumstances. The idea of writing a monograph was conceived in 1973, while I was Senior Lecturer in Pharmacology at Massey University, New Zealand. A large portion of the experimental data given in the book is the result of my own research, which was carried out mainly at The Ohio State University at Columbus. Most of the book was written in Columbus during 1976 and was completed in Western Australia. Far more distressing than the disruption caused by moving from one country to another is the token support and the frustration that I have experienced as a veterinary pharmacologist. I did intend to write a chapter on kinetics of the pulmonary uptake and the distribution of volatile anesthetics. Also, I would have liked to incorporate a number of solved examples and problems based on experimental data.

Emphasis is placed on the interpretation of data obtained following drug administration to animals, and I would like to point out that some of the views expressed are personal. Many of the drug translocation processes and pH gradient effects as well as principal metabolic pathways are supported by experimental data. Deficit of further suitable data precludes a greater number of illustrations of examples. The author hopes that this book will contribute to the scientific foundation on which the emerging discipline of veterinary clinical pharmacology can be developed. Although I intend to continue working at the basic level, I look to veterinary clinicians to apply the principles and to communicate their findings. The combined efforts of comparative pharmacologists and experienced veterinary clinicians should lead to more effective use of drugs in animals, with ultimate benefit to humans. The references supplied provide much valuable information and some, at least, should be consulted. A deliberate attempt was made to include what the author considers key articles among the references. Industrial veterinarians might find the information in this book helpful when designing experiments to determine drug residue profiles and to evaluate effectiveness of drug products.

I wish to thank Mr. Carroll Cann, Veterinary Editor, for his assistance and cooperation with the production of this book, and with whom it was indeed a pleasure to work. The precision and efficiency of Mrs. Laura Tarves, Mrs. Betty Richter and supporting staff at W. B. Saunders Company are gratefully acknowledged. I am indebted to Mrs. Arlene Myers for her accurate typing of the original manuscript. To my wife, Collete, and daughters, Siobhan and Jennifer, I with to express my sincere gratitude. Their understanding and patience with me appear to be infinite.

I would appreciate comments on the text, formulae and data presented, receipt of further references, or preferably reprints of articles, giving data on the absorption, distribution and elimination of drugs in domestic animals, and to be notified of any errors in the book. I shall endeavor to answer questions that readers may wish to pose.

J. DESMOND BAGGOT
Lesmurdie, Western Australia

Contents

1

General Principles Governing Translocation of Drugs

INTRODUCTION

Pharmacodynamics is the study of the biochemical and physiological effects of drugs, their mechanisms of action, and the factors that determine the intensity and temporal course of drug action in the body. A therapeutic agent may be defined as a drug which will produce a beneficial pharmacological or antimicrobial effect. Since drugs are potentially toxic chemicals, a therapeutic effect is likely to be obtained only when the drug is administered in proper dosage. The choice of therapeutic agent not only depends upon the effect desired, but also is influenced by the species of animal undergoing therapy. The clinician is responsible for administering a correct amount of drug in a suitable dosage form by an appropriate route. Certain drugs (e.g., anesthetic agents) are used to purposely alter normal functions. Inhalation anesthetic agents are not administered in predetermined doses but are regulated according to the observed depth of anesthesia.

The actions and effects of drugs on the various body systems are presented in textbooks of pharmacology. *The Pharmacological Basis of Therapeutics* (5th edition, edited by L. S. Goodman and A. Gilman)

1

and *Veterinary Pharmacology and Therapeutics* (4th edition, edited by L. E. McDonald and N. H. Booth) are comprehensive, modern and highly recommended. The *action* of a drug is defined as the process by which the chemical agent induces a change in some preexisting physiological function or biochemical process of the living organism. The location in the body at which the drug initiates the series of events (measured or observed as *effects*) that are produced by the drug is known as the *site of action*. The mechanism of action of most drugs is believed to involve a chemical interaction between the drug and a functionally important tissue component, called a receptor, in the living organism. The hypothetical receptor is regarded as a macromolecular tissue constituent with which a drug interacts to produce its characteristic biological effect (Ariëns and Simonis, 1964; Albert, 1968). Only the initial drug-receptor reaction is correctly termed the action of the drug; the succeeding events are properly called drug effects. It is axiomatic that no drug can cause a tissue to exert any response of which it is not naturally capable. The binding force that exists between a drug and its receptor arises from the concerted operation of several bond types. The drug-receptor combination usually involves ionic bonds, hydrogen bonds and Van der Waals forces; a reversible interaction is established, which obeys the law of mass action (Clark, 1937). Occasionally, stronger covalent bonds are formed and the drug effect is persistent and slowly reversed. The long-lasting inhibition of the cholinesterase enzymes by organic phosphates and carbamates is an example of drug-receptor interaction through formation of covalent bonds.

The aim of drug administration is to produce a desired clinical response (i.e., therapeutic effect), which most likely will be obtained by establishing and maintaining, for a certain period of time, an effective concentration of drug at its site of action. The size of the dose, route of administration, and bioavailability of the dosage form determine the amount of drug entering the bloodstream. For most therapeutic agents, there exists a range of plasma (or serum) drug concentrations at which effects of desirable intensity are achieved. The duration of action depends in a complex manner upon the relative rates of the various translocation processes and drug metabolic pathways. Absorption and distribution processes influence the drug concentration reached in the immediate vicinity of the receptor sites (biophase), whereas biotransformation (i.e., metabolism) and excretion terminate the action of a drug in the body. Comparison of the plasma concentration–time profiles obtained after intravenous administration of an anesthetic dose (25 mg/kg) of pentobarbitone to dogs and goats shows that the rates of disappearance of the unchanged drug from the blood plasma of the two species were very different (Fig. 1–1). The various reflexes (e.g., palpebral) returned and the

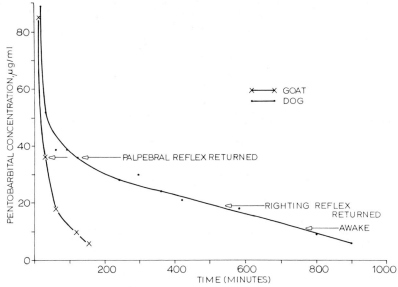

Figure 1–1 Concentrations of pentobarbitone in plasma of dogs and goats following intravenous administration of an anesthetic dose (25 mg/kg). Arrows indicate the plasma drug concentrations and related times at which reflexes returned. (From Davis, L. E., Neff-Davis, C. A., and Baggot, J. D. (1973): *In* L. T. Harmison (ed.): *Research Animals in Medicine*. Washington, D.C., U.S. Department of Health, Education, and Welfare, DHEW Publication No. (NIH) 72–333, pp. 715–732.)

animals of both species awakened at almost identical concentrations of drug in plasma. It was concluded that the species difference in duration of action of pentobarbitone is related to kinetic considerations rather than to differences in receptor sensitivity (Davis et al., 1973). An important point that must be mentioned is that plasma levels of unbound drug are related to pharmacological activity only when the action is rapidly reversible and metabolites of the drug are inactive.

Figure 1–2 illustrates how the various events (absorption, distribution and elimination) that constitute uptake and removal of drugs from the body are related. In order to achieve its effect, a suitable dosage form of the drug must be administered by an appropriate route. The drug in solution must then be absorbed from the site of administration. Upon entering the bloodstream, some of the drug molecules may bind reversibly to plasma proteins, usually albumin, and the remainder will undergo simultaneous distribution and elimination (i.e., biotransformation and excretion) processes. Passive diffusion is by far the most important mechanism for transfer of drug molecules across biological membranes. "Drug disposition" is a term used to

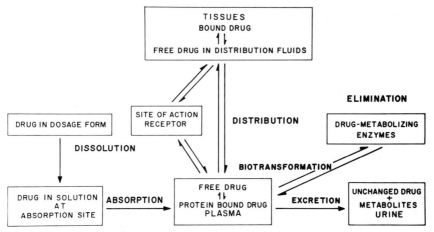

Figure 1–2 Schematic representation of the processes that influence uptake, access to site of action, and removal of a drug from the body.

describe the simultaneous effects of distribution and elimination. Distribution is usually a much more rapid process than elimination.

The pathways of biotransformation and routes of excretion constitute what is called the fate of a compound. The liver is the principal site of biotransformation, but drugs are also metabolized in other tissues. Metabolic alteration of structure is a prerequisite for excretion of many drugs. The kidney plays the major role in drug excretion except for volatile agents, such as inhalation anaesthetics, which are eliminated by the lungs. Drugs are sometimes given to produce local effects, in which case the aim is to minimize or delay absorption into the circulation; an example is the injection of a local anesthetic agent subcutaneously or into the spinal canal.

All the translocation processes of drugs, including access to the site of action, either directly or indirectly involve passage across biological membranes. It is essential, therefore, to review briefly the nature of membranes and the mechanisms of drug transport.

PASSAGE OF DRUGS ACROSS BIOLOGICAL MEMBRANES

Organization of Membranes

Membranes are the simplest example of molecules coming together to form a structural entity, but this structure may be sufficiently complex to attend to the specialized function of the membrane. Biological membranes may be viewed as mosaics of functional units composed of lipoprotein complexes (Dowben, 1969). Electron microscopic studies of tissues suggest that most membranes are composed of a fundamental structure called the unit membrane or plasma membrane. This boundary, which is 80 to 100 Å thick, surrounds single cells and nuclei. More complex barriers, such as the intestinal epithelium and the skin, are composed of multiples of this fundamental structure. The characteristic feature of cell membranes appears to be a bimolecular layer of phospholipid molecules, oriented perpendicular to the plane of the membrane, with polar head groups aligned at both surfaces, and long hydrocarbon chains extending inward (Davson and Danielli, 1952). It had been thought that sheets of "unfolded" protein molecules covered the inner and outer membrane surfaces, and that an additional layer of globular proteins (e.g., enzymes) was localized at the inner surface. However, more recent advances in electron microscopy and analytical data on membrane proteins have led to a different concept, the "fluid mosaic" model (Singer and Nicolson, 1972). In this model, the proteins that are integral to the membrane are a heterogeneous set of globular molecules, each arranged in an amphipathic structure, that is, with the ionic and highly

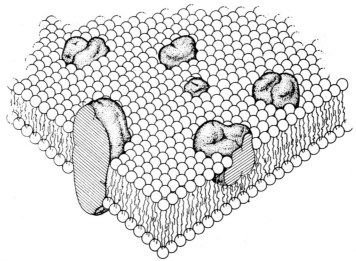

Figure 1–3 The lipid-globular protein mosaic model with a lipid matrix (the fluid mosaic model) of the cell membrane. The phospholipids are arranged as a discontinuous bilayer with their ionic and polar head groups (represented by the circles) in contact with water; the wavy lines represent the fatty acid chains. The solid bodies with stippled surfaces represent the globular integral proteins. The globular protein molecules are postulated to be amphipathic, as are the phospholipids. (From Singer, S. J., and Nicolson, G. L.: *Science, 175*:720–731, February 18, 1972. Copyright 1972 by the American Association for the Advancement of Science.)

polar groups protruding from the membrane into the aqueous phase, and the nonpolar groups largely buried in the hydrophobic interior of the membrane (Fig. 1–3). These globular molecules are partially embedded in a matrix of phospholipid. The bulk of the phospholipid is organized as a discontinuous, fluid bilayer, although a small fraction of the lipid may interact specifically with the membrane proteins. Aqueous channels appear to be present in the central axes of the globular integral proteins.

Drug Transport Across Membranes

Drug molecules pass across biological membranes either by passive transfer or by specialized transport processes (Schanker, 1964). In passive transfer processes, the membrane behaves as an inert lipoid-pore boundary, and drug molecules traverse this barrier either by diffusing through the lipoprotein region or by passing through the aqueous channels. Both nonpolar lipid-soluble compounds and polar water-soluble substances that possess sufficient lipid solubility can cross the predominantly lipoid plasma membrane by passive diffusion. The rate of penetration is directly proportional to the concentration gradient across the membrane and the lipid-to-water partition coefficient (i.e., lipid-solubility) of the drug. Passive diffusion is characterized by the movement of drug molecules down a concentration gradient without cellular expenditure of energy. Passage through channels is called filtration, since it involves bulk flow of water as a result of a hydrostatic or osmotic difference across the membrane. This bulk flow of water carries with it any water-soluble molecule that is small enough to pass through the channels. Filtration is a common mechanism for transfer of many small, water-soluble, polar and nonpolar substances. The apparent diameter of the aqueous channels differs in the various body membranes. The channels in the capillary membrane are large (40 to 80 Å depending on capillary location), while those in the intestinal epithelium and most cell membranes are about 4 Å in diameter. The capillary membrane is composed of an interlocking mosaic of endothelial cells separated by slits that could serve as pores. Although membrane permeability behavior suggests the presence of aqueous channels in biological membranes, electron microscopic confirmation of their presence is lacking, except in the arachnoid villi. Drug permeation through aqueous channels is of importance in renal excretion, removal of drugs from the cerebrospinal fluid, and passage of molecules across the liver sinusoidal membrane.

Most inorganic ions are sufficiently small to penetrate the pores in membranes, but their concentration gradients across the cell membrane are generally determined by the transmembrane potential (e.g., chloride ion) or by active transport (e.g., sodium and potassium ions).

The pH Partition Hypothesis

Most drugs are weak organic acids or bases and exist in solution as both the nonionized and the ionized forms. The nonionized molecules are usually lipid-soluble and readily cross the membrane to achieve the same equilibrium concentration on either side. In contrast, the ionized molecules are virtually excluded from transmembrane diffusion. Passage of an organic electrolyte across a biological membrane is therefore governed by the pH of the environment and the dissociation constant of the drug, since, according to the Henderson-Hasselbalch equation,

for an acid,

$$pH - pK_a = \log \frac{(\text{concentration of ionized acid})}{(\text{concentration of nonionized acid})} \qquad \textbf{Equation 1} \cdot \textbf{1}$$

and for a base,

$$pH - pK_a = \log \frac{(\text{concentration of nonionized base})}{(\text{concentration of ionized base})} \qquad \textbf{Equation 1} \cdot \textbf{2}$$

In these equations, the dissociation constant of both acids and bases is expressed as pK_a, which is the negative logarithm of the acid dissociation constant. The pK_a of a compound is a measure of its inherent acidity or alkalinity, and is determined by the molecular arrangement of the constituent atoms. From Equations 1·1 and 1·2 it can be seen that, when the pH and pK_a values are equal, 50 per cent of the drug is ionized and 50 per cent is nonionized. In the case of an acid, raising the pH of the solution increases the degree of ionization, and decreasing the pH decreases the degree of ionization (Table 1–1). The converse is true for bases. For an acid, increasing or decreasing the pH by one unit from the pK_a changes the degree of ionization to 90.9 per cent and 9.1 per cent, respectively. A change of the pH by two units changes the proportions to 99 per cent and 1 per cent. The majority of therapeutic agents have pK_a values between 3 and 11, and exist accordingly in both the nonionized and ionized forms within the range of physiological pH values. The quaternary ammonium compounds are an exception and exist in biological fluids only in the cationic form.

Table 1–1 INFLUENCE OF pH ON DEGREE OF IONIZATION (SHOWN AS PER CENT NONIONIZED) OF VARIOUS SULFONAMIDES

| | | | Per Cent Nonionized | | |
| | | | | PAROTID SALIVA | |
Sulfonamide	pK_a	PLASMA (pH, 7.4)	Human (6.4)	Horse (7.4)	Cow (8.4)
Sulfanilamide	10.4	99.9	100	99.9	99
Sulfapyridine	8.4	90.9	99	90.9	50
Sulfamethazine	7.4	50.0	90.9	50.0	9.1
Sulfadiazine	6.5	11.5	55.75	11.5	1.0
Sulfadimethoxine	6.0	3.85	28.6	3.85	0.4
Sulfacetamide	5.4	1.0	9.1	1.0	0.1

Per cent nonionized $= 100 - \dfrac{100}{1 + 10^{(pK_a - pH)}}$

$10^{(pK_a - pH)}$ is antilog $(pK_a - pH)$

Since diffusion is the mechanism for passage of drugs across biological membranes, one would expect no further net transmembrane movement when the concentrations of nonionized drug become the same on both sides of the membrane. However, when a pH gradient exists across the membrane, unequal concentrations (nonionized plus ionized) of the drug will be attained on either side; at equilibrium, there will be a higher total concentration of drug on the side of the membrane where the degree of ionization is greater. This mechanism is known as ion trapping. The partitioning of a weak acid (pK_a 4.4) between plasma (pH 7.4) and gastric juice (pH 1.4) is illustrated in Figure 1–4. It is assumed that the gastric mucosal membrane behaves as a simple lipoid barrier which is permeable only to the nonionized form of the acid. At equilibrium, the total (nonionized plus ionized) drug concentration ratio between plasma and gastric juice will be ap-

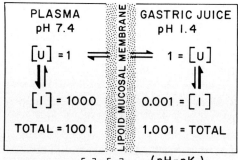

WEAK ACID $[I] = [U] \cdot 10^{(pH - pK_a)}$

Figure 1–4 Influence of pH on the distribution of a weak acid between plasma and gastric juice, which are separated by a lipoid barrier. In this figure, [I] and [U] represent the concentrations of the ionized and nonionized forms of the drug, respectively. It is assumed that the gastric mucosal membrane is permeable only to the nonionized form of the compound.

proximately 1000:1. This ratio would be reversed for a weak base with a pK_a of 4.4. Acidic drugs (e.g., salicylates, sulfonamides) attain higher concentrations in the relatively more alkaline body fluids. Basic drugs (e.g., narcotic analgesics, the antiarrhythmic agents quinidine, procainamide and lidocaine) readily enter and tend to concentrate in the more acidic fluids, including the intracellular fluids (pH 7.0). Applications of this phenomenon, the pH partition hypothesis, are widespread. Weak organic acids are rapidly and well absorbed from the stomachs of dogs and cats. Likewise, the acidic urinary reaction found in carnivorous species promotes passive reabsorption of acidic drugs, with pK_a values between 3.0 and 7.2, from the distal portion of the nephron. Weak organic bases, administered parenterally, diffuse passively into ruminal fluid (pH 5.5 to 6.5) of cattle and sheep, where they become trapped by ionization and exposed to the metabolic action of microorganisms. Weak acids may enter ruminal fluid by way of alkaline saliva (pH 8.0 to 8.4). The flow of mixed saliva in cows fed in different ways was estimated to lie between 98 and 190 liters during a 24 hour period (Bailey, 1961). The daily secretion in sheep was estimated at 6 to 16 liters (Kay, 1960). While ruminants secrete saliva constantly, horses do so only during mastication (Alexander, 1966). The saliva of the horse is nearly neutral (pH 7.3 to 7.6) in reaction, and the daily secretion of parotid saliva is probably of the order of 10 to 12 liters. For comparison, humans secrete 1 to 1.5 liters of a hypotonic saliva, poorly buffered and usually slightly acidic (Schmidt-Nielsen, 1946; Eastoe, 1961).

The theoretical equilibrium concentration ratio ($R_{x/y}$) of a drug on opposite sides of a biological membrane may be calculated, on the basis of the degree of ionization of the electrolyte, according to the following equations (Jacobs, 1940):

for an acid,

$$R_{x/y} = \frac{1 + 10^{(pH_x - pK_a)}}{1 + 10^{(pH_y - pK_a)}}, \text{ or} \qquad \text{Equation 1 \textbullet 3}$$

$$R_{x/y} = \frac{1 + \text{antilog}(pH_x - pK_a)}{1 + \text{antilog}(pH_y - pK_a)}$$

and for a base,

$$R_{x/y} = \frac{1 + 10^{(pK_a - pH_x)}}{1 + 10^{(pK_a - pH_y)}}, \text{ or} \qquad \text{Equation 1 \textbullet 4}$$

$$R_{x/y} = \frac{1 + \text{antilog}(pK_a - pH_x)}{1 + \text{antilog}(pK_a - pH_y)}$$

For both weak acids and weak bases the total concentration of drug is greater on the side of the membrane where it is more highly ionized. One should be aware that, while the pH partition hypothesis usually provides a good approximation of the distribution of a weak organic electrolyte between the water phase of blood plasma (or serum) and another biological fluid, it cannot be considered so seriously that it is used to postulate that biological barriers are generally impermeable to ions, and to attribute observed deviations from its predictions to thermodynamically untenable mechanisms that invoke a "virtual pH" (Smolen, 1973). In many instances, equilibrium is never achieved, either because the drug diffuses from a small volume into a much larger volume or because it is rapidly removed by elimination; the diffusion process is then unidirectional.

An unequal distribution of drug across a membrane can also exist at equilibrium if there is a difference in the extent of protein (or other macromolecule) binding on either side of the membrane. Protein-bound drug molecules, like ionized molecules, cannot permeate cellular membranes. Thus, at equilibrium there will be a higher total concentration of drug on the side of the membrane at which the greater extent of binding occurs.

Passage of Antimicrobial Agents into Milk

The parenchyma of the mammary gland is organized into a multicompartment organ with aggregations of alveoli partitioned off into lobules by thin connective tissue septa. The lobules, drained by a common collecting duct, form a lobe, and the lobes in turn make up the gland. Histological sections of the mammary glands of different species are quite similar. The walls of the secretory portions (the alveoli and the finer ducts) consist of a basal lamina, a layer of myoepithelial cells and, on the internal surface of the resting gland, a single layer of low columnar epithelial (glandular) cells. During lactation the shape of the glandular cells fluctuates from cylindrical or conical to flat. Milk is a suspension of fat droplets in an aqueous phase in which lactose, inorganic salts, and proteins, mainly casein, are dissolved.

Studies of the penetration of antimicrobial agents from the systemic circulation into milk indicate that the mammary gland epithelium behaves as a lipoidal membrane which separates blood of pH 7.4 from milk, which has a somewhat lower pH value (normal pH range is 6.5 to 6.8). The passage of each drug into milk is determined by the extent of binding to plasma albumin, the pK_a value and the degree of lipid solubility. The binding of antibiotics in bovine serum varies very considerably (Ziv and Sulman, 1972). Although oxytetracycline is

only 20 per cent bound to serum proteins, the longer-acting derivatives metacycline, doxycycline and minocycline are extensively
bound (80 to 90 per cent) at similar concentrations of the drugs.
Among the penicillins, cloxacillin is highly bound (about 75 per cent),
phenethicillin, phenoxymethylpenicillin, and benzylpenicillin are moderately bound (35 to 65 per cent), whereas ampicillin is only 18 per
cent bound to serum proteins. Within the therapeutic range (0.1 to
10 μg/ml), the percentage of penicillin bound is independent of the
penicillin concentration (Keen, 1965). In contrast, the extent of binding of cephalexin is concentration-dependent; about a sevenfold
increase in the percentage binding (from 3 per cent to 22.4 per cent)
was found as the concentration of cephalexin in serum decreased
from 16.2 to 0.5 μg/ml (Ziv and Sulman, 1972). Chloramphenicol,
erythromycin, lincomycin, tylosin and trimethoprim are bound between 25 and 50 per cent, while the aminoglycosides streptomycin,
gentamicin, kanamycin and spectinomycin occur predominantly free
in blood plasma, being less than 13 per cent bound to proteins. Binding of sulfonamides to bovine plasma proteins (albumin) varies with
the compound and, within the therapeutic range of plasma levels (50
to 150 μg/ml), the percentage bound tends to decrease with increasing
sulfonamide concentration, although the total amount of drug bound
increases with increasing concentration (Fig. 1–5). The percentage
binding of various sulfonamide compounds to bovine plasma pro-

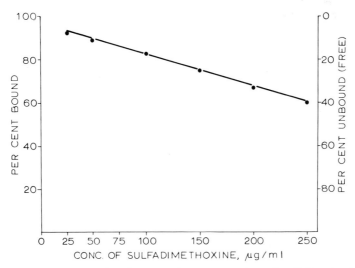

Figure 1–5 Relationship between the concentration of sulfadimethoxine in
bovine plasma and the percentage bound to the proteins. Extent of binding at each
concentration of the drug was measured by equilibrium dialysis at 37°C using blood
plasma collected from six normal cows.

Table 1-2 BINDING OF SULFONAMIDES TO
BOVINE PLASMA PROTEINS
(TOTAL SULFONAMIDE CONCENTRATION IN PLASMA WAS 100 μg/ml)

Compound	Per Cent Bound	Reference
Sulfadimethoxine	83	Stowe and Sisodia, 1963
Sulfisoxazole	76	Anton, 1960
Sulfamethoxypyridazine	66	Anton, 1960
Sulfadimidine	65	
Sulfadiazine	24	Anton, 1960
Sulfanilamide	22	

teins, presumably albumin, at a total sulfonamide concentration of 100 μg/ml, is tabulated in Table 1-2.

It has been shown that only the lipid-soluble, nonionized moiety of an organic electrolyte in the water phase of blood plasma diffuses into milk (Rasmussen, 1966). The binding of sulfonamides to milk proteins varies from zero to 40 per cent depending on the derivative. In normal lactating cows, weak acids give milk ultrafiltrate–to–plasma ultrafiltrate concentration ratios less than or equal to 1; weak bases, excluding aminoglycoside antibiotics, attain concentration ratios greater than 1 (Table 1-3). The limited extent of penetration of the aminoglycoside antibiotics into milk can be related to their extremely

Table 1-3 PASSAGE OF CHEMOTHERAPEUTIC AGENTS FROM
THE SYSTEMIC CIRCULATION INTO MILK

Drug	pK$_a$	Milk pH	Concentration Ratio (Milk Ultrafiltrate: Plasma Ultrafiltrate) THEORETICAL	EXPERIMENTAL	Reference*
Organic Acids:					
Benzylpenicillin G	2.7	6.8	0.20	0.13–0.26	Ziv et al., 1973 b
Cloxacillin		6.8	0.20	0.25–0.30	Ziv et al., 1973 b
Ampicillin		6.8	0.26	0.24–0.30	Ziv et al., 1973 b
Cephaloridine	3.4	6.8	0.25	0.24–0.28	Ziv et al., 1973 b
Sulfadimethoxine	6.0	6.6	0.19	0.23	Stowe and Sisodia, 1963
Sulfamethazine	7.4	6.6	0.55	0.59	Rasmussen, 1958
Organic Bases:					
Tylosin	7.1	6.8	3.0	3.5	Ziv and Sulman, 1973 a
Lincomycin	7.6	6.8	2.83	2.50–3.60	Ziv and Sulman, 1973 b
Trimethoprim	7.6	6.5–6.8	2.8–5.3	2.90–4.90	Rasmussen, 1970
Erythromycin	8.8	6.8	6.1	8.7	Rasmussen, 1959
Kanamycin	(7.8)	6.5–6.9		0.60–0.80	Ziv and Sulman, 1974

*The individual references should be consulted for the design of each experiment. It is important to know the method of drug administration, as after a single intravenous injection equilibrium will never be established.

poor solubility in nonpolar solvents and to their low lipid-to-water partition coefficients. Since the passage of most antimicrobial agents from the systemic circulation into milk is in accordance with the pH partition hypothesis and the milk-to-plasma concentration ratios for acids and bases can be predicted by Equations 1·3 and 1·4, respectively, it follows that a change in the pH of milk will influence the drug level produced in the milk. For weak organic bases, the milk-to-plasma concentration ratio of total drug will decrease with increasing pH of milk (Table 1–4). Consequently, lower milk levels of antibiotics that are bases will be attained in cows affected with mastitis (milk pH reaction may be increased up to 0.7 of a pH unit) than in normal lactating animals. The choice of antimicrobial agent for systemic therapy of mastitis should be based upon the susceptibility of the infecting microorganism to the drug, and upon the milk drug level which may be attained with usual dosage. The former can be determined *in vitro,* and the latter may be predicted.

Passage of Drugs into the Central Nervous System

A drug may enter the tissue of the central nervous system (CNS) by two distinct routes: the capillary circulation and the cerebrospinal

Table 1–4 PASSAGE OF ORGANIC BASES INTO MILK

Drug	pK$_a$	Milk pH	Concentration Ratio (Milk Ultrafiltrate: Plasma Ultrafiltrate)		Reference
			THEORETICAL	EXPERI-MENTAL	
Tylosin	7.1	6.5	4.98	5.2	Ziv and Sulman, 1973 *a*
		6.8	3.00	3.5	
		7.1	1.00	1.0	
Lincomycin	7.6	6.5	5.42	5.5	Ziv and Sulman, 1973 *b*
		6.8	2.83	3.05	
		7.1	1.16	2.65	
Clindamycin	7.7	6.5	5.61	6.2	Ziv and Sulman, 1973 *b*
		6.8	2.98	3.7	
		7.1	1.66	2.2	
Chloramphenicol		6.5–6.8		1.1	Ziv et al., 1973 *a*
		7.1		1.1	
Spectinomycin	8.75	6.5	7.66	0.5*	Ziv and Sulman, 1973 *a*
		6.8	4.24	0.6	
		7.1	2.00	0.7	

*Passage of spectinomycin into milk was limited by its high degree of ionization in serum (95.8 per cent) and its low lipid-solubility.

fluid (CSF). In a pharmacological sense, the extracellular fluid (ECF) of the brain and the cerebrospinal fluid act as if they were intracellular fluids (Rall et al., 1959). The probability of drug access to the brain and cerebrospinal fluid resembles that of drug entry into the intracellular fluid of typical somatic cells, such as muscle cells. It should be pointed out, however, that any compound that is present in the blood will enter the tissues of the central nervous system to a certain, if very limited, extent.

The capillaries of the brain are unlike the porous capillaries in muscle and most other tissues; their endothelial cells are joined one to another by continuous tight intercellular junctions. These junctions appear to represent complete apposition of the neighboring cell membranes. In addition, certain cells within the brain connective tissue (the astrocytes) have long processes which form sheaths that are in close approximation to the capillary endothelium. Accordingly, drug molecules in plasma must diffuse through the endothelial cells and the astrocytic sheath in order to reach the brain extracellular fluid (Fig. 1–6). The permeability characteristics of brain capillaries are similar to those of somatic cell membranes. The "blood-brain barrier" allows only unbound lipid-soluble drug molecules in blood plasma to enter (by passive diffusion) the extracellular fluid of brain tissue. Because of the high cerebral blood flow — about 16 per cent of the cardiac output — drugs that are highly lipid-soluble enter the central ner-

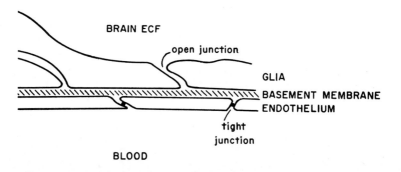

Figure 1–6 Schematic representation of the blood-brain barrier. The extracellular fluid of the brain is separated from blood plasma by the cerebral parenchymal capillaries and a surrounding cuff of glial tissue. Tight junctions occlude intercellular clefts of the vascular endothelium; clefts between astrocytic end-feet are open, connecting the endothelial basal lamina (or basement membrane), which does not seem to be a barrier, with brain extracellular fluid. For a drug to diffuse from plasma into extracellular fluid of the brain it must pass through the capillary endothelium, but may then move within the intercellular clefts between processes of the glial investment. (From Cserr, H., Fenstermacher, J. D., and Rall, D. P. [1970]: In B. Schmidt-Nielsen and D. W. S. Kerr [eds.]: Urea and the Kidney. Amsterdam, Excerpta Medica, pp. 127–137.)

CSF

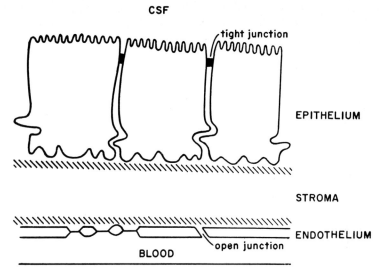

tight junction

EPITHELIUM

STROMA

ENDOTHELIUM

open junction

BLOOD

Figure 1–7 Schematic representation of the choroid plexus. The cerebrospinal fluid is separated from blood plasma by the tissue of the choroid plexus. Intercellular clefts of the vascular endothelium appear to be open; tight junctions, however, connect adjacent choroidal epithelial cells. For a drug to enter cerebrospinal fluid from blood, it can move within the open junctions between capillary endothelial cells, but it must pass through the choroidal epithelial cells. (From Cserr, H., Fenstermacher, J. D., and Rall, D. P. [1970]: *In* B. Schmidt-Nielsen and D. W. S. Kerr [eds.]: *Urea and the Kidney*. Amsterdam, Excerpta Medica, pp. 127–137.)

vous system quite rapidly. The inhalation anesthetic agents (e.g., diethyl ether, halothane, methoxyflurane) are compounds of diverse structure, but they all possess high lipid-solubilities and readily enter the tissues of the central nervous system.

The cerebrospinal fluid is formed by a process of active secretion, largely by the choroid plexus of the lateral, third and fourth ventricles (Davson, 1967). It flows through the ventriculocisternal system, bathes the surfaces of the brain and spinal cord (subarachnoid space), and then flows into the venous blood sinuses through a system of large channels and valves in the arachnoid villi (Welch and Friedman, 1960). In the choroid plexus the capillary endothelial cells have open junctions (i.e., the usual porous structure). However, the choroidal epithelial cells are joined to one another with continuous tight junctions. Consequently, the transfer of chemical substances from the blood across the choroid plexus into the cerebrospinal fluid has the characteristics of passage across epithelium, since the drug must pass through the choroidal cells (Fig. 1–7). The functional membrane, which only lipid-soluble drug molecules in plasma water can traverse to enter cerebrospinal fluid, is referred to as the "blood-CSF barrier."

The pH of CSF is normally about 0.1 unit more acid than plasma (Rall et al., 1959). This would favor the slight concentration in CSF of weak organic bases. Lipid-soluble drug molecules that are free (not bound to proteins) in blood plasma, in general, enter the extracellular fluid of the brain and cerebrospinal fluid at about the same rate. Should a concentration gradient exist between the two fluids, the drug will passively diffuse across the ependyma from the fluid of higher drug concentration to that of lower concentration. Drugs leave the brain by diffusion and the CSF by bulk flow into the venous blood sinuses and diffusion into capillaries. If the compound is an organic electrolyte, it may be removed from CSF by an active carrier-mediated transport process (analogous to that in the proximal renal tubule) at the choroidal epithelial cells (Rall and Sheldon, 1961). Penicillin is an example of an organic acid which is actively removed from CSF at the choroid plexus. Penicillin (pK_a 2.7) is a water-soluble cyclic peptide bearing a carboxyl group that is completely ionized at plasma pH. What little enters the brain ECF and the CSF penetrates the blood-brain and blood-CSF barriers very slowly, except in meningeal infections, when penetration into CSF may be increased.

Passage of Barbiturates into the Cerebrospinal Fluid

The barbiturates, a group of weak organic acids that enter cerebrospinal fluid from blood, have a combination of physicochemical properties that favor passive diffusion across the blood-CSF barrier. A low degree of ionization at plasma pH and fairly high lipid-solubility of the nonionized moiety are properties that confer ready penetration of a compound into cerebrospinal fluid. It is only the lipid-soluble, nonionized molecules in the water phase of blood plasma that can diffuse through the choroidal epithelial cells. The rate of penetration of a barbiturate into CSF is determined mainly by the degree of lipid-solubility of the compound (Table 1–5). Thiopentone (pK_a 7.6) passes into the cerebrospinal fluid very rapidly owing to the extremely high lipid-solubility of the nonionized molecules. The concentrations of thiopentone in plasma water and cerebrospinal fluid of a dog given a single dose (25 mg/kg) of the drug are shown in Figure 1–8. Equilibration apparently occurred within 5 min of the dose. Although the plasma level declines rapidly because of distribution into all the tissues, the drug moves out of the CSF and brain to maintain equilibrium. The ultrashort duration of action of thiopentone following rapid intravenous injection of a single dose of the drug is a consequence of its high lipid-solubility, because this property confers upon it the ability to enter and leave the CNS very rapidly. The low

Table 1–5 CORRELATION OF PHYSICAL PROPERTIES OF
SOME BARBITURATES WITH THEIR RATES OF PENETRATION
INTO CEREBROSPINAL FLUID*

(a) Drug	(b) Fraction Bound to Plasma Protein at pH 7.4	(c) pK$_a$	(d) Fraction Nonionized at pH 7.4	(e) Partition Coefficient n-Heptane/H$_2$O of Nonionized Form	(f) Effective Partition Coefficient, (d) × (e) (×10^3)	(g) Penetration Half-time (min)
Thiopental	0.75	7.6	0.613	3.3	2000	1.4
Pentobarbital	0.40	8.1	0.834	0.05	42	4.0
Barbital	<0.02	7.8	0.715	0.002	1.4	27.0

*Data from Brodie, B. B., et al. (1960): The importance of dissociation constant and lipid-solubility in influencing the passage of drugs into the cerebrospinal fluid. *J. Pharmacol. exp. Ther.,* *130*:20–25. © 1960, The Williams and Wilkins Company, Baltimore.

blood supply to fat depots (about 2 per cent of cardiac output) re-stricts rapid uptake of the drug into body fat. Most of a single dose eventually becomes localized in fat depots, from which tissue the drug is released very slowly and then eliminated (Fig. 1–9). Pentobarbitone (pK$_a$ 8.1), the oxygen homologue of thiopentone, is less ionized in plasma but has a much lower partition coefficient, and therefore pene-trates the blood-CSF barrier more slowly. The onset of anesthesia takes 2 to 3 min, and the duration of the anesthetic effect is 3 to 4 hours in dogs given a single anesthetic dose of pentobarbitone. The technique of inducing anesthesia with this drug, which involves introducing about

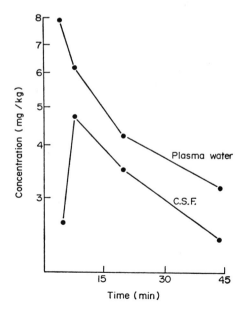

Figure 1–8 Concentrations of thiopentone in plasma water and cerebrospinal fluid of a dog given an intravenous dose of 25 mg/kg. (From Brodie, B. B., Bernstein, E., and Mark, L. C. [1952]: *J. Pharmacol. exp. Ther.,* *105*:421–426.)

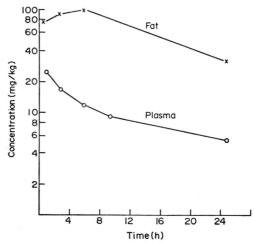

Figure 1–9 Concentrations of thiopentone in plasma and fat (lumbodorsal region) of a dog after the intravenous administration of 25 mg/kg. (From Brodie, B. B., Bernstein, E., and Mark, L. C. [1952]: *J. Pharmacol. exp. Ther., 105*:421–426.)

two thirds of the dose calculated to be necessary rapidly into the bloodstream, followed by increments of the remainder at short intervals "to effect," is based on the rate of its penetration into the central nervous system. Pentobarbitone is eliminated by the hepatic microsomal enzyme systems, and the inactive metabolites are excreted in urine. Barbitone (pK$_a$ 7.8) is considerably less bound to plasma proteins than thiopentone and a higher fraction is nonionized in plasma, but it penetrates the blood-CSF barrier very slowly, owing to its very low degree of lipid-solubility. The slow onset of action renders this drug useless as an anesthetic or hypnotic agent. Phenobarbitone (pK$_a$ 7.3) has a relatively low lipid-solubility and enters the CNS slowly, but it is a useful anticonvulsant agent when given orally to dogs in proper dosage.

Specialized Transport Processes

Specialized transport processes appear to be responsible for the rapid cellular transfer of certain foreign organic ions and polar molecules, as well as many natural substrates, such as sugars, amino acids and pyrimidines. These processes give the cell membrane the flexibility and selectivity it requires to control the movement of specific substances into and out of the cell. Specialized transport is generally thought to be mediated by carriers (that is, membrane components that form a reversible complex with the substance to be transported.) Two types of carrier-mediated transport can be distinguished—namely, facilitated diffusion and active transport (Wilbrandt and Rosenberg, 1961; Stein, 1967). Competitive inhibition is characteristic of carrier-mediated transport. Specialized transport processes differ from passive transfer in that the former exhibit relative selectivity and saturability, and active transport requires the direct expenditure of energy. Active transport is responsible for the rapid transfer into urine and bile of unchanged molecules of many organic electrolytes, as well as the polar metabolites of the majority of drugs, and is involved in the removal of certain drug molecules from the central nervous system at the choroid plexus and ciliary body; to a lesser extent, it is also involved in the intestinal absorption of compounds structurally related to some dietary constituents. The transported substance is transferred against a concentration or electrochemical gradient (uphill transport). Facilitated diffusion, like passive diffusion, requires no further expenditure of cellular energy, and movement occurs only with the concentration gradient. This type of transport is responsible for the rapid transfer of glucose and amino acids across membranes of various cells. The transport of glucose across the gastrointestinal mucosa and by the kidney, however, is an active process and can proceed against a concentration gradient. For drugs, there is evidence, although it is inconclusive, to suggest that facilitated diffusion processes may exist for the transport of some water-soluble agents.

Pinocytosis is a transport mechanism which, like active transport, requires the expenditure of cellular energy. It differs from active transport in that transfer of the solute is mediated not by combination with a carrier but by the local invagination of the cell membrane and subsequent budding off within the cell interior of a vesicle that contains the solute (Lewis, 1931; Fawcett, 1965). Pinocytotic uptake of colloidal particles, viruses, macromolecules and other materials that are readily adsorbed onto cell surfaces involves several features which are characteristic of carrier-mediated transport generally—notably selectivity (although apparently of a low order), competition and saturation kinetics (Gosselin, 1967). The capacity of the newborn calf to absorb soluble protein molecules from colostrum is attributed to occurrence of pinocytosis. Pinocytotic activity may be responsible for transcapillary passage of macromolecules and uptake of solutes by pulmonary alveolar epithelial cells. The pinocytotic process might be initiated by the binding of an extracellular macromolecule onto the cell surface, and it appears that the size and charge of the macromolecule are important factors in determining its degree of uptake (Chapman-Andresen, 1964; Fawcett, 1965; Ryser, 1968).

Water and small-sized lipid-insoluble molecules may traverse aqueous channels, but ultrafiltration and bulk flow are important processes for the translocation of drugs only at sites where the plasma membrane has been specially modified to accommodate these processes (e.g., renal glomeruli, arachnoid villi).

REFERENCES

Albert, A. (1968): *Selective Toxicity*. 4th Ed. London, Methuen, p. 68.

Alexander, F. (1966): A study of parotid salivation in the horse. *J. Physiol.* (Lond.), *184*:646–656.

Anton, A. H. (1960): The relation between the binding of sulfonamides to albumin and their antibacterial efficacy. *J. Pharmacol. exp. Ther., 129*:282–290.

Ariëns, E. J., and Simonis, A. M. (1964): A molecular basis for drug action. *J. Pharm. Pharmacol., 16*:137–157.

Bailey, C. B. (1961): Saliva secretion and its relation to feeding in cattle. III. The rate of secretion of mixed saliva in the cow during eating, with an estimate of the magnitude of the total daily secretion of mixed saliva. *Brit. J. Nutr., 15*:443–451.

Brodie, B. A., Bernstein, E., and Mark, L. C. (1952): The role of body fat in limiting the duration of action of thiopental. *J. Pharmacol. exp. Ther., 105*:421–426.

Brodie, B. B., Kurz, H., and Schanker, L. S. (1960): The importance of dissociation constant and lipid-solubility in influencing the passage of drugs into the cerebrospinal fluid. *J. Pharmacol. exp. Ther., 130*:20–25.

Chapman-Andresen, C. (1964): Measurement of material uptake by cells: pinocytosis. *In* D. M. Prescott (ed.): *Methods in Cell Physiology*. Vol. 1. New York, Academic Press, pp. 277–304.

Clark, A. J. (1937): *In* A. Heffter (ed.): *Handbuch der Experimentellen Pharmakologie*. Supplement IV. General Pharmacology. Berlin, Springer-Verlag. p. 63.

Cserr, H., Fenstermacher, J. D., and Rall, D. P. (1970): Permeabilities of the choroid plexus and blood-brain barrier to urea. *In* B. Schmidt-Nielsen and D. W. S. Kerr (eds.): *Proceedings of the International Colloquy on Urea and the Kidney*. Amsterdam, Excerpta Medica, pp. 127–137.

Davis, L. E., Neff-Davis, C. A., and Baggot, J. D. (1973): Comparative pharmacokinetics in domesticated animals. *In* L. T. Harmison (ed.): *Research Animals in Medicine*. Washington, D.C., U.S. Department of Health, Education, and Welfare. Publication No. (NIH) 72–333, pp. 715–732.

Davson, H. (1967): *Physiology of the Cerebrospinal Fluid*. London, Churchill.

Davson. H.. and Danielli, J. F. (1952): *The Permeability of Natural Membranes*. 2nd Ed. London, Cambridge University Press, pp. 57–71.

Dowben, R. M. (1969): Composition and structure of membranes. *In* R. M. Dowben (ed.): *Biological Membranes*. Boston, Little Brown, pp. 1–38.

Eastoe, J. E. (1961): The chemical composition of saliva. *In* C. Long (ed.): *Biochemists' Handbook*. Princeton, Van Nostrand, p. 907.

Fawcett, D. W. (1965): Surface specializations of absorbing cells. *J. Histochem. Cytochem., 13*:75–91.

Gosselin, R. E. (1967): Kinetics of pinocytosis. *Fed. Proc., 26*:987–993.

Jacobs, M. H. (1940): Some aspects of cell permeability to weak electrolytes. *Cold Spring Harbor Symp. Quant. Biol., 8*:30–39.

Kay, R. N. B. (1960): The rate of flow and composition of various salivary secretions in sheep and calves. *J. Physiol.* (Lond.), *150*:515–537.

Keen, P. M. (1965): The binding of three penicillins in the plasma of several mammalian species as studied by ultrafiltration at body temperature. *Brit. J. Pharmacol., 25*:507–514.

Lewis, W. H. (1931): Pinocytosis. *Johns Hopk. Hosp. Bull., 49*:17–27.

Rall, D. P., and Sheldon, W. (1961): Transport of organic acid dyes by the isolated choroid plexus of the spiny dogfish, *S. acanthias. Biochem. Pharmacol., 11*:169–170.

Rall, D. P., Stabenau, J. R., and Zubrod, C. G. (1959): Distribution of drugs between blood and cerebrospinal fluid: general methodology and effect of pH gradients. *J. Pharmacol. exp. Ther., 125*:185–193.

Rasmussen, F. (1958): Mammary excretion of sulfonamides. *Acta Pharmacol. Toxicol., 15*:139–148.

Rasmussen, F. (1959): Mammary excretion of benzylpenicillin, erythromycin, and penethamate hydroiodide. *Acta Pharmacol. Toxicol., 16*:194–200.

Rasmussen, F. (1966): *Studies on the Mammary Excretion and Absorption of Drugs.* Copenhagen, Carl Fr. Mortensen.

Rasmussen, F. (1970): Renal and mammary excretion of trimethoprim in goats. *Vet. Rec., 87*:14–18.

Ryser, H. J.-P. (1968): Uptake of protein by mammalian cells: an underdeveloped area. *Science, 159*:390–396.

Schanker, L. S. (1964): Physiological transport of drugs. *In* N. J. Harper and A. B. Simmonds (eds.): *Advances in Drug Research.* Vol. 1, New York, Academic Press, pp. 71–106.

Schmidt-Nielsen, B. (1946): The pH of parotid and mandibular saliva. *Acta physiol. scand., 11*:104–110.

Singer, S. J., and Nicolson, G. L. (1972): The fluid mosaic model of the structure of cell membranes. *Science, 175*:720–731.

Smolen, V. F. (1973): Misconceptions and thermodynamic untenability of deviations from pH-partition hypothesis. *J. pharm. Sci., 62*:77–79.

Stein, W. D. (1967): *The Movement of Molecules Across Cell Membranes.* New York, Academic Press, pp. 1–35.

Stowe, C. M., and Sisodia, C. S. (1963): The pharmacologic properties of sulfadimethoxine in dairy cattle. *Am. J. vet. Res., 24*:525–535.

Welch, K., and Friedman, V. (1960): The cerebrospinal fluid valves. *Brain, 83*:454–469.

Wilbrandt, W., and Rosenberg, T. (1961): The concept of carrier transport and its corollaries in pharmacology. *Pharmacol. Rev., 13*:109–183.

Ziv, G., and Sulman, F. G. (1972): Binding of antibiotics to bovine and ovine serum. *Antimicrob. agents Chemother., 2*:206–213.

Ziv, G., and Sulman, F. G. (1973a): Serum and milk concentrations of spectinomycin and tylosin in cows and ewes. *Am. J. vet. Res., 34*:329–333.

Ziv, G., and Sulman, F. G. (1973b): Penetration of lincomycin and clindamycin into milk in ewes. *Brit. vet. J., 129*:83–91.

Ziv, G., and Sulman, F. G. (1974): Distribution of aminoglycoside antibiotics in blood and milk, *Res. vet. Sci., 17*:68–74.

Ziv, G., Bogin, E., and Sulman, F. G. (1973a): Blood and milk levels of chloramphenicol in normal and mastitic cows and ewes after intramuscular administration of chloramphenicol and chloramphenicol sodium succinate. *Zbl. Vet.-Med., A., 20*:801–811.

Ziv, G., Shani, J., and Sulman, F. G. (1973b): Pharmacokinetic evaluation of penicillin and cephalosporin derivatives in serum and milk of lactating cows and ewes. *Am. J. vet. Res., 34*:1561–1565.

2

The Absorption of Drugs; Bioavailability

INTRODUCTION

In order for a drug to act and exert its characteristic systemic effects, it must be absorbed and attain an effective concentration at its site of action. An increasing body of information tends to support the hypothesis that drug effect, therapeutic or toxic, is more closely correlated with plasma concentration than with dose (Levy, 1968a). Drug absorption is usually defined as the passage of a drug from its site of administration into the bloodstream. Most drugs are administered as drug products, not as drug entities.* The biological performance of a drug product can be affected by its bioavailability, which is defined as the rate and extent to which a drug administered as a drug product enters the systemic circulation in an unchanged form. Absorption of drugs is governed by the route of administration, the dosage form, and certain physicochemical characteristics of the compound. A drug in solution will probably be well absorbed if it is lipid-soluble, if it is not completely ionized and if its molecular weight is not excessively high (Keberle, 1971).

The possible routes of drug entry into the body may be divided into two classes: enteral and parenteral. In enteral administration the

---

*"Drug product" means a prepared dosage form (e.g., tablet, capsule, solution) that contains the active drug ingredient, generally but not necessarily in association with inactive ingredients.

22

drug is placed directly in the gastrointestinal tract; parenteral administration implies that the gastrointestinal tract is bypassed. Thus, oral
doses are enteral, and injection, topical application to the skin and
inhalation by the lungs are all parenteral routes. Absorption is dependent upon drug solubility, regardless of the site of administration.
Drugs given in aqueous solution are more rapidly absorbed than those
given in oily solution, suspension or solid form. For drugs given in
solid dosage form (tablet, capsule, suspension), the rate of dissolution
may be the limiting factor in their absorption. The concentration of a
drug also influences its rate of absorption. Other factors which are important determinants of the rate of drug absorption are the area of the
absorbing surface to which a drug is exposed, and blood supply to the
site of absorption.

PARENTERAL ADMINISTRATION

Parenteral routes of administration include intravenous (I.V.), intramuscular (I.M.) and subcutaneous (S.C.) injections when a systemic effect is desired, and tissue infiltration, intra-articular and
epidural injections when a localized action is sought. Parenteral therapy necessitates that strict asepsis be maintained. Gaseous and volatile liquid anesthetic agents may be inhaled and are rapidly absorbed
into the systemic circulation by diffusing across the pulmonary alveolar epithelium. These drugs all have relatively high lipid-to-water
partition coefficients, are of small atomic or molecular radii and are
absorbed over extensive surfaces richly supplied with blood, so that
they all equilibrate nearly instantaneously with blood in the alveolar
capillaries. The interesting differences among these agents in the kinetics of their equilibration in body water and in the rates of onset
and decline of their anesthetic effects depend primarily upon their
aqueous solubilities (blood-to-air partition coefficients). The pulmonary alveolus is lined with a single layer of flat epithelial cells, forming
an extremely thin barrier between the alveolar air and the interstitium, which is richly supplied with capillaries. The alveolar epithelium
and capillary wall are so closely associated that the total air-blood
barrier is only 0.5 to 1 μm thick. Solutions of drugs can be atomized
and the fine droplets in air (aerosol) can then be inhaled. In pulmonary disease, this technique of drug administration achieves local
application of the drug at the site of infection and almost instantaneous
absorption into the circulation. Its main disadvantages are poor ability
to regulate the dose and possible irritation of the mucous membranes
of the respiratory tract. Topical application and intramammary infusion are routes of drug administration employed when local effects

are sought; a variable degree of absorption, which depends on physicochemical properties of the drug and the vehicle, takes place from these sites of application.

Intravenous Injection

The injection of a drug solution directly into the bloodstream gives a predictable concentration of the drug in plasma and produces an extremely rapid pharmacological response. Another advantage of the intravascular route is control over the rate of introduction of drug into the general circulation. In some instances, as in the induction of surgical anesthesia with pentobarbitone, the exact dose of the drug is not predetermined but is adjusted to the response of the animal. In healthy dogs, about two-thirds of the computed probable dose (28 mg/kg) is injected rapidly as soon as venipuncture has been performed, in order to ensure that the dog passes smoothly through the second (i.e., narcotic excitement) stage of anesthesia. The remainder of the computed dose is administered in increments and "to effect." In feeble animals or those with toxic reactions the speed of injection must be quite slow from the commencement, for not infrequently it is found that half the calculated normal dose produces deep anesthesia in such animals (Hall, 1971). Intravenous infusion is a satisfactory method of maintaining therapeutic plasma concentrations of drugs that have short half-lives and relatively narrow margins of safety. Complete bioavailability of a drug is assured only when the intravascular route of administration is employed. Biophasic availability is generally reserved for situations in which pharmacological data are used to assess biological performance (Smolen, 1971). The rapid introduction into the bloodstream of a small dose of thiopentone as a single I.V. bolus is a special application of the intravenous technique. The aim of this procedure, in horses premedicated with a phenothiazine ataractic drug (e.g., acetylpromazine), is to induce anesthesia of short duration, enabling the operator to insert an endotracheal tube so that a longer period of anesthesia can be instituted and maintained wth an inhalation agent (e.g., halothane). The ultrashort duration of the anesthetic effect produced by the rapid intravenous injection of a small dose of thiopentone is a consequence of the very high lipid-solubility of the nonionized drug moiety (61 per cent) in the plasma water; this property enables the drug molecules to enter and leave the tissues of the central nervous system very rapidly.

Although the intravenous route has many advantages, it is potentially the most dangerous route of drug administration and great care must be exercised in computing the total dose to be administered and in controlling the rate of injection. In drug therapy, single I.V. doses must always be given slowly, ideally over a period of time approximately equal to a complete circulation of the blood. In intravenous infusions as much attention must always be given to both the amount of drug and the volume of fluid administered per minute. Because of all the attendant dangers, the intravenous route of administration for a drug should be selected only after all the alternatives have been considered and rejected.

Absorption from Intramuscular
and Subcutaneous Sites

Intramuscular and subcutaneous administration of drugs can result in absorption rates very different from those obtained after oral administration. The capillary endothelial tissue forms a barrier against drug entry into the systemic circulation. The rates at which all substances penetrate endothelial tissue at various sites except the brain are far in excess of those at which these same compounds cross epithelial tissue. The rate of absorption of drugs from aqueous solutions depends mainly on the vascularity of the injection site, but other factors include the degree of ionization and lipid-solubility of organic electrolytes, molecular size of lipid-insoluble substances, and the area over which the injected solution has spread (Schou, 1961; Sund and Schou, 1964). Absorption of most drugs from aqueous solutions injected intramuscularly or subcutaneously is relatively rapid; the peak concentration in plasma (or serum) is usually reached within one-half to 1 hour. A drug may influence its own rate of absorption and the uptake of another drug administered simultaneously if it alters the blood supply or capillary permeability at the site of injection. Addition of epinephrine (1 part in 200,000) (Scott et al., 1972) or other vasoconstrictor (e.g., vasopressin) to a solution of local anesthetic agent (e.g., procaine) will prolong the duration of local analgesia beyond that produced by administration of the anesthetic agent alone.

Intramuscular injection of single doses of gentamicin and kanamycin in dogs and ketamine in cats showed that these drugs were completely available systemically. The assumption that all drugs injected intramuscularly and subcutaneously are completely *bioavailable* is, however, invalid, as was found for intramuscularly administered diazepam (Gamble et al., 1973), digoxin (Greenblatt et al., 1973), and phenytoin (formerly diphenylhydantoin) (Wilensky and Lowden, 1973). Whereas the sodium salt of cephalexin is poorly absorbed after intramuscular injection (Gower et al., 1973; Nicholas et al., 1973), the lysine salt of cephalexin is well absorbed (Barrios et al., 1975). The greater solubility of the latter and the better buffering capacity of lysine probably account for this difference in systemic availability of the drug from the two cephalexin salts in muscle tissue. Dosage forms of ery- thromycin (injectable) and tylosin (base in 50 per cent propylene glycol) intended for intramuscular injection in cows give low levels of antibiotic activity in serum, which persist for some hours. The slow absorption from these drug products determines the level and duration of serum antibiotic activity. Drugs that are relatively insoluble at tis- sue pH or that are dissolved or suspended in an oily vehicle form a depot in muscle tissue, from which small fractions of the dose are avail- able for absorption over an extended period. The principal reason for using depot preparations is to reduce the frequency of dosage. Pro- longed levels of penicillin activity in serum can be achieved by the in- tramuscular injection of procaine penicillin suspended in oil containing aluminum stearate. An effective way of achieving extremely slow ab- sorption is to incorporate a drug into a compressed pellet that can be implanted subcutaneously. The drug must be quite insoluble and the pellet must resist disintegration by the subcutaneous fluid environment. Certain steroid hormones (e.g., desoxycorticosterone acetate, estradiol and testosterone) have been incorporated into pellets; these drugs are highly insoluble. It has been hypothesized that, in order to achieve a constant rate of absorption, the ideal shape for a pellet for subcutane- ous implantation is a flat disc.

Certain drug solutions (e.g., 33 per cent [330 mg/ml] sodium sul- famethazine) are too irritant to tissue and cause severe pain when in- jected subcutaneously, probably because the pH lies outside the physiological range of values. These drug solutions may, however, be administered by slow intravenous injection.

Percutaneous Absorption

The transfer of foreign compounds from the outer surface of the skin through the keratin layer *(stratum corneum)* and cells of the epidermis and the dermis, and from here into the bloodstream, is known as percutaneous absorption. The major route for skin penetra- tion of foreign compounds is via the closely adherent epidermal cells. The efficacy of a dermatological preparation is directly related to the ability of the drug to penetrate the skin barrier. It has been shown that the barrier to skin permeability is the stratum corneum, and that individual compounds show different permeability characteristics, depending on their own particular properties of solubility and dif- fusion (Schuplein, 1965; Schuplein and Blank, 1971). After topical application of a dermatological preparation to the surface of the skin, the active drug must dissolve, be released from the vehicle, and begin to accumulate in the keratin layer. The stratum corneum is a heterogeneous tissue composed of flattened keratinized cells. However, when the drug transfers to the granular layer *(stratum granulosum)* it readily reaches the local sites of action. The rate-limiting step, which controls the overall process of percutaneous absorption, can be the rate of dissolution, the release from the vehicle residue, or transfer into and through the keratin layer (Riegelman, 1974). As soon as the drug enters the bloodstream it is distributed throughout the body and undergoes biotransformation and excretion. This route of drug administration, like the I.M. and S.C. routes, avoids exposure of the intact molecule to the metabolic effects of the liver before entering the systemic circulation ("first-pass effect").

The barrier properties of the skin vary with the site of application and with the species of animal. Species differences in skin penetration following topical application of a radiolabeled organophosphorus compound to isolated skin sections are shown in Table 2-1.

The efficacy of dosage forms for topical drugs is often dependent on the composition of the vehicle. The ability of a topical preparation of a drug to penetrate the skin and exert its effect is dependent on two consecutive physical events. The drug must diffuse out of the vehicle to the skin surface, and it must then penetrate this natural barrier en route to the site of action. Many so-called "vehicle effects" reported in the literature are consequences of these two diffusional processes. Depending on which process proceeds more slowly, either event could determine the overall effectiveness of the topical dosage form. These two processes are intimately related, and both are dependent on the physical properties of the drug, the vehicle, and the barrier.

Table 2-1 MAXIMAL PENETRATION OF RADIOLABELED ORGANOPHOSPHORUS COMPOUND THROUGH EXCISED SKIN FROM DORSAL THORAX OF VARIOUS SPECIES*

Species	Rate (μg/cm^2/min)
Pig	0.3
Dog	2.7
Monkey	4.2
Goat	4.4
Cat	4.4
Guinea pig	6.0
Rabbit	9.3
Rat	9.3

*Data from McCreesh, A. H. (1965): *Toxicol. appl. Pharmacol.*, 7(Suppl. 2):20-26.

The percutaneous absorption of drugs from vegetable oils and animal fats that tend to penetrate through the skin is superior to that from mineral oils (Eller and Wolf, 1939; Harry, 1941; Valette, 1953). The effects of various oily vehicles on the percutaneous absorption of salicylic acid (pK_a 3.0) was studied by measuring the amount of the drug excreted in the urine; the drug was substantially absorbed from lard and lanolin, but only slightly absorbed from petrolatum (Bourget, 1893; Kimura, 1940).

When a skin infection is located in the deeper layers of the epidermis or in the dermis, systemic therapy with antibacterial or antifungal agents is often more effective than topical application. Mycotic disease of the skin, hair and nails from *Microsporum, Trichophyton* or *Epidermophyton*, for example, responds well to oral therapy with griseofulvin. Owing to the insolubility of griseofulvin in aqueous media, absorption from the intestine is very poor in humans; the micronized preparations are much better absorbed. It must be stressed that, since other fungal diseases are not affected by the drug, careful mycological study with identification of the responsible organism is the only basis on which therapy can be selected accurately.

Various agents have been reported as sorption promoters, such as the hydrophilic solvent propylene glycol or surfactants. However, the most effective accelerants are aprotic materials such as dimethyl sulfoxide, dimethylformamide and dimethylacetamide. On application to the skin, dimethyl sulfoxide passes rapidly through the stratum corneum (Stoughton, 1965; Allenby et al., 1969), and has been found, in vivo, to accelerate the penetration through the skin of water (Baker, 1968), fluocinolone acetonide (Stoughton and Fritsch, 1964), salicylic acid (Kligman, 1965), and other substances. Dimethyl sulfoxide can also establish a reservoir in the stratum corneum of compounds with low water-solubility and to which the epidermis is only slightly permeable (Munro and Stoughton, 1965). Anionic surfactants (e.g., sodium lauryl sulfate) increase the skin penetration of water-soluble substances, possibly because of their ability to increase the permeability of the skin to water.

Since the skin is a biological barrier and chemical agents penetrate by passive diffusion, it is not surprising that excessive exposure to highly lipid-soluble substances, such as organic phosphate insecticides and organic solvents, can cause serious toxic effects. The skin barrier is vulnerable to certain solvents and organic amines, as reflected by sharp increases in skin permeability (Vinson et al., 1965). There is greater penetration of drugs through damaged skin than through intact skin. Particular care should be taken when considering application of topical preparations to cats because they groom themselves by licking.

ADMINISTRATION OF DRUGS
BY THE ENTERAL ROUTE

The most common route of administration of drugs is by mouth (orally, per os, P.O.). In general, absorption takes place along the entire length of the gastrointestinal tract, but the small intestine is the principal site for absorption of most drugs. The gastrointestinal mucosa has the properties of a lipoidal barrier endowed with aqueous pores and has, in addition, a number of enzyme or carrier systems that are responsible for the transport of water-soluble nutrient molecules. The mechanism for absorption of organic electrolytes is passive nonionic diffusion, which depends essentially on the movement of lipid-soluble drug molecules across the mucosa and into the bloodstream down a concentration gradient. The physicochemical properties of each drug determine the extent and principal site of absorption (Brodie and Hogben, 1957). The low degree of ionization and high lipid-solubility (lipid-to-water partition coefficient) of the nonionized moiety are properties favorable to the absorption of organic electrolytes. According to the pH partition hypothesis, weakly acidic drugs are mainly nonionized and lipid-soluble in acid solution and should, therefore, be well absorbed from the stomach of humans and monogastric animals, such as the dog, cat and pig. Weakly basic drugs should be absorbed from the less acidic (or more alkaline) contents (pH 6.6) of the small intestine. An effective pH of 5.3 in the microenvironment of the absorbing surface of the intestinal epithelial barrier appears to determine the degree of ionization and extent of absorption of organic electrolytes. Detailed studies with a large number of drugs in unbuffered solutions revealed that in the normal intestine weak acids with pK_a values above 3 and bases with pK_a values of less than 7.8 are very well absorbed; outside these limits the absorption of both acids and bases diminished rapidly (Hogben et al., 1959). The absorption of strong organic acids and bases and quaternary ammonium compounds is generally poor and variable, since ionization is virtually complete over the whole range of physiological pH. Drugs do not seem to be absorbed via the small intestinal lymphatics to any significant extent. Although most drugs and other foreign compounds cross the intestinal barrier by passive diffusion, there is evidence that a foreign compound can be absorbed by a specialized transport process if its chemical structure closely resembles a nutrient that is actively absorbed.

Glucose and amino acids are transported across the intestinal wall by specific carrier systems. Ionic iron is absorbed as an amino acid complex, at a rate usually determined by the body's need for iron (Bothwell, 1968). Sodium ion is probably transported actively across the intestinal wall. Magnesium ion is very poorly absorbed, and when administered orally as a salt (e.g., magnesium sulfate) will act as a cathartic, retaining an osmotic equivalent of water as it moves along the intestinal tract.

There is often marked individual variation in the response obtained after oral administration of a drug product; slow or incomplete absorption is probably a common but rarely recognized cause of therapeutic failure in clinical practice. Most oral dosage forms are solids (e.g., capsules and tablets). Absorption of a drug from the gastrointestinal tract involves release of the drug from its dosage form (unless the latter is a solution) and access to and transfer across the mucosal barrier into the hepatic portal venous blood. The term "dosage form" includes the chemical nature (salt or simple derivative), physical state (amorphous or crystalline, solvated or nonsolvated, and so forth), and the particle size, distribution and surface area of the drug itself in the dosage form. Drug release from a tablet involves disintegration and dissolution. Dissolution is usually complete for most drug substances, but may cause variation in the rate of release of the active compound from the product. When drugs are administered as tablets, suspensions or capsules, release from the dosage form is frequently rate-limiting for the overall absorption process (Levy, 1968b). Occasionally dissolution, especially of sparingly soluble drugs, is so protracted that it controls not only the absorption process but also the overall rate of elimination of the drug from the body. Dissolution can be enhanced by using the salt form of a drug (e.g., potassium phenoxymethyl penicillin, phenytoin sodium, propranolol hydrochloride, promazine hydrochloride) or by decreasing the particle size (e.g., spironolactone, griseofulvin), thereby increasing bioavailability of the therapeutic agent. Drug absorption from a suspension is usually more rapid than from a tablet.

Even when a drug product is completely dissolved, many factors can influence its bioavailability. A drug in solution will probably be well absorbed if it is lipid-soluble, not completely ionized and stable (i.e., neither chemically nor enzymatically inactivated) in the gastrointestinal fluids. Penicillin G and erythromycin, for example, are unstable in the acidic gastric fluids; chloramphenicol is inactivated by ruminal microorganisms. During the process of absorption, drug molecules are exposed to enzymes in the intestinal mucosa, and molecules absorbed from the stomach and small intestine are conveyed in hepatic portal blood to the liver (which is the principal site of biotransformation for most drugs) before reaching the general circulation. Biotransformation by enzymes in the gut mucosa or the liver, or both, may significantly reduce bioavailability of orally administered drugs, particularly if metabolism is extensive, as was found with lidocaine (Boyes et al., 1970), propranolol (Dollery et al., 1971), imipramine (Gram and Christiansen, 1975), and nortriptyline (Alexanderson et al., 1973; Gram and Overø, 1975). To distinguish between intestinal and hepatic metabolism, a drug must be introduced in a manner that bypasses the gastrointestinal tract—such as by direct infusion into the hepatic portal vein or, perhaps, by intraperitoneal administration. At the present time, however, intraperitoneal administration must be considered with reservations. The effect of biotransformation preceding drug entry into the systemic (or general) circulation ("first-pass effect") would be similar to, and could be misinterpreted as, incomplete absorption. The amount of drug lost depends on the rate of absorption, activity of enzymes in the intestinal mucosa and the hepatic extraction ratio, which is that fraction of the drug entering the liver that is cleared by elimination processes.

Since the absorptive capacity of the small intestine is so much greater than that of the stomach (because of the extensive surface area and rich blood supply of the mucosa), gastric emptying time is a critical determinant of the overall absorption rate of drugs, regardless of whether they are weak acids, weak bases or neutral compounds. The rate of gastric emptying depends on various physiological factors, such as autonomic and hormonal activity, and on the volume and composition of the gastric contents. The absorption rate of a drug administered in solid dosage form is determined mainly by dissolution of the drug product, but it is also influenced by physicochemical characteristics of the drug and blood flow to the intestine.

As indicated earlier, drug solutions injected intraperitoneally (I.P.) are absorbed primarily into the portal venous blood and, therefore, must pass through the liver before entering the systemic circulation (Lukas et al., 1971).

Comparative Aspects of Drug Absorption

The domestic animals may be divided, on the basis of dietary habits, into herbivorous (horse, ox, sheep and goat), omnivorous (pig) and carnivorous (dog and cat) species. The pH gradients between plasma and the gastrointestinal fluids of the various species play an important role in determining the extent of absorption of orally given drug products, and degree of distribution or excretion into the gastrointestinal tract of parenterally administered weak organic electrolytes.

The physiology of digestion and drug absorption processes are, in general, similar in the dog, cat and pig, and are not unlike those in the human. The gastric juice is highly acid (pH 1 to 2) in these species, whereas the intestinal contents are nearly neutral, but actually slightly acid. Although the stomach is a significant site of absorption for many weak acids and neutral compounds, the upper small intestine is the most important site of absorption for all orally administered drug products. The rate of gastric emptying, therefore, markedly influences the absorption of drugs.

It is difficult to appreciate the functions of the stomach of the adult horse. Under normal conditions of feeding this organ is never empty, and the pH of its contents has been observed to vary from 1.13 to 6.8 (Schwarz et al., 1926). Evidence exists that substantial amounts of lactic acid are produced in the equine stomach as a result of bacterial fermentation, and most of this acid appears to be absorbed in the small intestine, thus contributing to the nutrition of the horse (Alexander, 1972). The parotid saliva, which has a high bicarbonate concentration (about 50 mEq/liter), may be the principal factor controlling the fermentation process. Parotid saliva is secreted only during mastication. Another distinguishing feature of the equine digestive tract is the adaptation of the large intestine to microbial digestion of polysaccharides.

The characteristic feature of the ruminant animal is the anatomical structure of the anterior portion of its alimentary canal. The rumen, reticulum and omasum, collectively called the forestomachs, are lined with a stratified squamous epithelium, which is keratinized in its outer layer. The approximate capacities of the adult reticulorumen are 100 to 225 liters in cattle and 6 to 20 liters in sheep and goats. The reticulorumen never empties, and its contents are of a semisolid consistency and are acidic (pH 5.5 to 6.5) (Annison and Lewis, 1959). Despite the stratified squamous nature of its epithelial lining, the rumen has been shown to have considerable absorptive capacity (Phillipson and McAnally, 1942; Danielli et al., 1945; Gray, 1948; Masson and Phillipson, 1951). The principal feature of digestive physiology in the ruminant animal is that continuous fermentation takes place in the reticulorumen, a large diverticulum in the gut between the esophagus and the abomasum (the stomach which secretes gastric juice). The herbage the host consumes is mixed with saliva and delivered to the fermentation organ (reticulorumen), whose musculature agitates the contents by highly organized waves of contraction. After comminution of the contents by both microbial digestion and rechewing, the more fluid portion is pumped by the omasum, an organ with filtering and absorptive capabilities, into the abomasum. Thereafter the digestive functions follow the familiar pattern of animals with a single stomach. The acidity of abomasal contents does not vary very much and usually remains close to pH 3 (Masson and Phillipson, 1952). Drug products given orally to ruminant animals must dissolve in reticuloruminal fluid and always undergo considerable

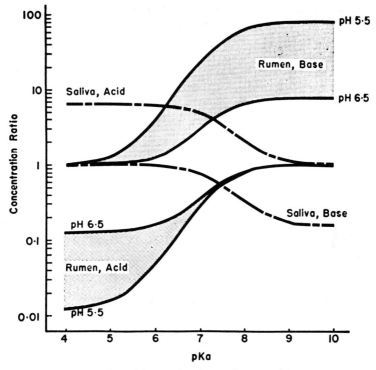

Figure 2–1   Expected equilibrium distribution between saliva or rumen contents and plasma of acids and bases of differing pKa. Concentration ratio is the ratio of the salivary or ruminal concentration to concentration free in the plasma, calculated separately for acids and bases, for saliva of pH 8.2 and rumen contents over a range of pH 5.5 to 6.5, assuming plasma is pH 7.4. (From Dobson, A. [1967]: *Fed. Proc., 26*:994–1000.)

dilution in this organ. The ruminal microflora may inactivate certain drugs by metabolic transformations of a hydrolytic or reductive nature. The concentration of a weak organic electrolyte in ruminal fluid, which is not metabolized by the microorganisms, will normally reflect the activities of both salivary and ruminal epithelial processes (Fig. 2–1). Passage of weak organic bases by nonionic diffusion from blood plasma into ruminal fluid, with subsequent ionization therein (ion trapping), is an important aspect of the disposition of such drugs in ruminant species.

BIOAVAILABILITY

Bioavailability refers both to the rate of drug absorption and to the extent (or completeness) of absorption. By extent of absorption is meant the fraction *(F)* of the oral or intramuscular dosage form which reaches the systemic circulation intact. To determine extent of absorption (i.e., fraction available systemically), an intravenous dosage study must also be performed. The product of the fraction available systemically and the administered dose *(F · D)* is called the "absorbed dose." Bioavailability is but the first of many factors that determine the relation between drug dosage and intensity of action.

Extent of Drug Absorption

For the purposes of most bioavailability studies, it is sufficient to determine three indices on a graph: the maximum concentration of drug reached in plasma (peak of plasma concentration–time curve), the time at which the peak concentration is present, and the area under the plasma drug concentration–time curve (Fig. 2–2). The peak plasma level is dependent on both the extent and the rate of drug absorption. The time at which the plasma drug concentration reaches its maximum is closely related to the absorption rate. It must be pointed out, however, that drug absorption continues after the peak plasma concentration has been reached. The usual method for estimating the extent of absorption *(F)* involves comparison of the total areas under

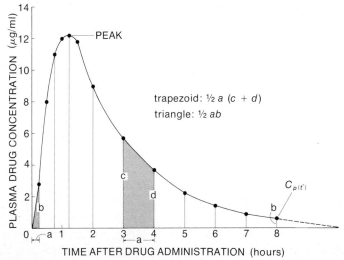

Figure 2–2 Trapezoidal method for estimating area under the curve (AUC). The total area under a curve (plotted on arithmetic coordinates) may be estimated by adding together areas of the trapezoids and triangle at each end of the curve. A better estimate of the area under the tail of the curve than that based on the extrapolated triangle is given by $C_{p(t^*)}/\beta'$, where $C_{p(t^*)}$ is the last measured concentration of drug in the plasma and β' is the apparent overall elimination rate constant obtained from the terminal slope of the semilogarithmic plot of the plasma drug concentration-time profile (see Equation 6·26). A maximum drug level of 12.2 µg/ml was present in plasma at 1.25 hours. The value of $C_{p(t^*)}$ is 0.6 µg/ml ($t^* = 8$ hours); $\beta' = 0.462$ hour^{-1} (from semilogarithmic plot). The area under the curve is closely related to the amount of drug that enters the systemic circulation intact.

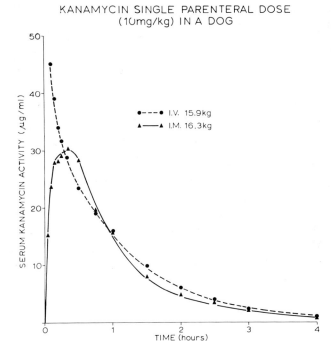

Figure 2–3   Concentrations (activity) of kanamycin in serum of a dog after intra-venous and intramuscular dosage (10 mg/kg) of the drug. The systemic availability of kanamycin from this product, based on comparison of the areas under the curves and taking into account the value of β for each route of administration, was 94 per cent.

the (linear) plasma level versus time curves obtained after oral (or other route) and intravenous administration of equal doses of the drug to the same animals. The area is measured by an appropriate numeri-cal integration procedure, and is expressed as the product of concen-tration and time. The curves which depict the change in serum kanamycin activity with time, plotted on arithmetic (linear) coordin-ates after intramuscular and intravenous dosage (10 mg/kg) of the drug in a dog, are shown in Figure 2–3. Inspection of the curve after intramuscular dosage shows that a peak serum kanamycin activity of 30.5 μg/ml was present at 20 min. The systemic availability of kanamycin after intramuscular dosage was obtained by comparing the areas under the curves, which were calculated according to the trapezoidal rule:

$$F = \frac{(\text{AUC})_{\text{I.M.}}}{(\text{AUC})_{\text{I.V.}}} = \frac{(\int_0^\infty C_P dt)_{\text{I.M.}}}{(\int_0^\infty C_P dt)_{\text{I.V.}}}$$

Equation 2•1

where $\int_0^\infty C_P dt = \int_0^{t^*} C_P dt + \dfrac{C_{P(t^*)}}{\beta}$

An estimate of the infinite part of the curves was obtained from $C_{P(t^*)}/\beta$, where $C_{P(t^*)}$ was the last measured concentration of the drug and β the overall elimination rate constant. To improve the estimate of F, the area under the curve was multiplied by the apparent overall elimination rate constant of the drug after dosage by the same route—i.e., $(AUC)_{I.M.} \times \beta^1/(AUC)_{I.V.} \times \beta$. This correction takes care of intrasubject variability in the overall elimination rate constant (β) of the drug. Kanamycin was found to be completely available systemically ($F \simeq 90$ per cent) when a single dose (10 mg/kg) of the drug product (5 per cent aqueous solution of kanamycin sulfate [Kantrim]*, 50 mg/ml) was given to six dogs by intramuscular injection. Gentamicin was also found to be completely available systemically in dogs when a single intramuscular dose (10 mg/kg) of gentamicin sulfate in aqueous solution (Gentocin†, 50 mg/ml) was administered.

The systemic availability of kanamycin after intramuscular and intratracheal administration of single doses (10 mg/kg) of the same drug product (Kantrim, 200 mg/ml) to a sheep were 100 per cent and 38 per cent, respectively. The curves of serum kanamycin activity versus time, plotted on arithmetic coordinates, are shown in Figure 2–4. It may be concluded that whereas the intramuscular route of kanamycin administration would produce therapeutically effective

*Kantrim, Bristol Laboratories, Syracuse, New York.
†Gentocin, Schering Corporation, Kenilworth, New Jersey.

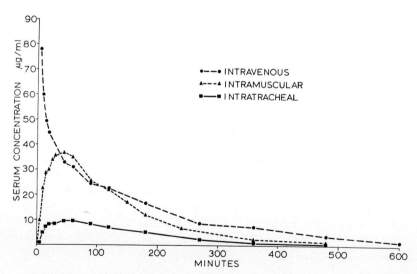

Figure 2–4   Concentration-time profiles of serum kanamycin (activity) in a sheep after administration of intravenous, intramuscular, and intratracheal doses (10 mg/kg) of the same drug product (Kantrim).

Table 2–2   BIOAVAILABILITY OF SOME DRUG PRODUCTS IN
DOMESTIC ANIMALS

Drug Product	Dose (mg/kg)	Species of Animal ($n = 6$)	Route of Administration	Systemic Availability* (per cent)	Peak Serum Level	
					TIME (min)	AVERAGE CONCENTRATION (μg/ml)
Ketamine hydrochloride	25	Cat	I.M.	92	10	12
Ampicillin trihydrate	10	Cat	S.C.	56	60	15
Sulfadimethoxine (suspension)	55	Dog	Oral	50	180–270	67
Kanamycin sulfate	10	Dog	I.M.	90	15–30	28
Gentamicin sulfate	10	Dog	I.M.	>90	30	30
Kanamycin sulfate	10	Horse	I.M.	>90	60–90	30
Digitoxin (tincture)	0.066	Dog	Oral	90	90–180	0.022
Tylosin (in 50% propylene glycol)	12.5	Cow	I.M.	70–80	360 ± 120	0.85
Erythromycin	12.5	Cow	I.M.	70–80	600 ± 300	1.00
Salicylate (aspirin tablets)	50	Cow	Oral	50–70	150	22
	100					45

*These values should not be considered absolute.

serum levels of the antibiotic, the intratracheal injection of this drug product would be unsatisfactory for systemic therapy.

The extent (or completeness) of drug absorption is always clinically important. The systemic availabilities of some drug products in domestic animals are tabulated in Table 2–2. The data presented in this table clearly show that rapid and complete access of a drug to the systemic circulation cannot be assumed *a priori* unless the drug is injected directly into the vascular system. It must be pointed out that although a drug product may have a relatively high systemic availability, a slow rate of absorption from the site of administration may give subtherapeutic plasma (or serum) levels of the drug. Administration of usual doses of such a drug product will give the impression that the drug is ineffective. This may be an erroneous conclusion, since adjustment of the dose or modification of the drug product may be all that is needed to make therapy effective. The slow absorption rates of tylosin (tylosin base in 50 per cent propylene glycol) and erythromycin (injectable) from intramuscular sites of administration yield subtherapeutic levels in serum (< 1.0 μg/ml) for the majority of potentially susceptible microorganisms (Fig. 2–5). Owing to a suitable combination of physicochemical properties (degree of lipid-solubility, extent of ionization), therapeutically effective levels of these macrolide antibiotics may be obtained in milk (Fig. 2–6).

When a drug product shows poor systemic availability, it becomes necessary to distinguish between dosage form and physiolog-

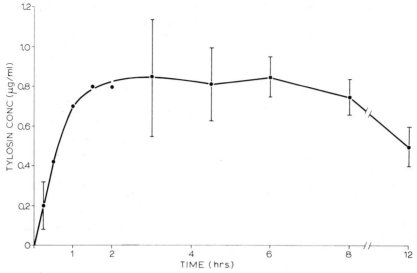

Figure 2–5 Tylosin concentrations (mean ± S.D.) in serum of cows ($n = 6$) after intramuscular injection of tylosin base in 50 per cent propylene glycol at a dose of 12.5 mg/kg body weight.

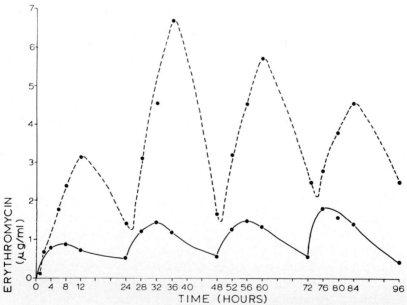

Figure 2–6 Erythromycin concentrations (activities) in serum (•———•) and milk (•— —•) after intramuscular dosage (12.5 mg/kg) of the antibiotic at 24 hour intervals. Each point shown is the mean concentration obtained in samples collected at that time from three cows.

ically modified bioavailability, which includes drug absorption interactions. Biotransformation by enzymes in the intestinal mucosa or liver, or both, preceding drug entry into the systemic circulation ("first-pass effect") may significantly reduce the bioavailability of an oral dosage form, despite favorable dissolution and absorption properties. A change from one brand of drug to another can result in therapeutic failure or unexpected toxicity, owing to differences in systemic availability of the drug from the various products.

The systemic availability of a drug from a number of drug products can be compared by obtaining cumulative urinary excretion data after administration of a single dose by any route. It is essential, however, that the fate of the drug be known and its form in urine (unchanged drug or major metabolite) be quantifiable. Although one would normally recommend a urinary collection period of seven times the half-life value of the drug, there is evidence that a shorter collection period may be adequate. Digoxin is excreted unchanged in the urine of humans. Even though an average of only 47 per cent of the 6 day cumulative urinary digoxin excretion was recovered in the first 24 hours, this urinary collection period is sufficient for comparative single-dose studies of systemic availability (Greenblatt et al., 1974). Griseofulvin has an average half-life of 11 to 14 hours (Rowland et al., 1968; Chiou and Riegelman, 1971), and the major urinary metabolite is 6-desmethylgriseofulvin (free and glucuronide conjugate). Systemic availability of griseofulvin from various commercial products of the drug can be assessed adequately from 24 hour total 6-desmethylgriseofulvin urinary excretion data (Bates and Sequeira, 1975).

Rate of Drug Absorption

Although some idea of the absorption rate of a drug in a particular dosage form can be derived from the time at which the maximum concentration is present in plasma, exact information on absorption rates of drugs in domestic animals is almost nonexistent in the literature. The Wagner-Nelson (1964) and Loo-Riegelman (1968) equations are extremely useful methods for calculating absorption rates of drugs. Both methods, however, require knowledge of the disposition kinetics of the drug in the animals being treated, which can only be determined after rapid intravenous injection of single doses. The choice as to which equation is the more appropriate for a particular drug depends upon the relative values of the individual rate constants that describe distribution and elimination of the drug after intravenous dosage. When the rate of distribution considerably exceeds that of elimination, the Wagner-Nelson equation may be employed. In all other situations, the Loo-Riegelman equation will yield the more correct answer. In a recent article, a potential source of error in absorption rate calculations was described (Boxenbaum and Kaplan, 1975). From either equation, per cent drug absorbed–time data can be generated. These methods place no limitation on the order of the absorption rate process. However, semilogarithmic plots of per cent remaining to be absorbed versus time frequently are linear and yield an apparent first-order absorption rate constant (k_{ab}).

The mean plasma level–time curves, plotted on arithmetic coordinates, obtained after administration of single doses (55 mg/kg) of 10 per cent sodium sulfadimethoxine solution intravenously and 12.5 per cent sulfadimethoxine suspension orally to six beagles weighing 9.0 to 11.0 kg are shown in Figure 2–7. The median systemic availability of sulfadimethoxine from the oral product, based on comparison of the areas under the plasma level–time curves after oral and intravenous dosage, was 32.8 per cent (range, 22.5 to 80.0 per cent). The areas were calculated by the trapezoidal rule and systemic availability was determined for each animal.* Inspection of the mean curve obtained

---

*When correction was made for intrasubject variability in β, the more accurate estimate of F gave a higher median value (48.8 per cent; range, 24.4 to 86.2 per cent) for systemic availability of the drug product.

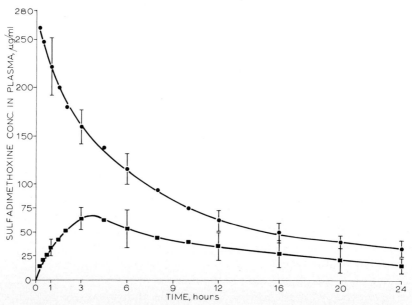

Figure 2–7 Concentrations (mean ± S.D.) of sulfadimethoxine in the plasma after administration of a fixed dose (55 mg/kg) by the intravenous (•) and oral (■) routes to a group of six dogs. The drug products administered were the injection (10 per cent) and oral suspension (12.5 per cent). (From Baggot, J. D., Ludden, T. M., and Powers, T. E. [1976]: *Can. J. comp. Med.*, 40:310–317.)

after oral dosage shows that a maximum concentration of 67 µg/ml was present in plasma at 3.6 hours. The distribution half-time (2.50 ± 0.45 hours) and half-life (13.21 ± 2.20 hours) of sulfadimethoxine were obtained from the intravenous study. The rate constant of absorption after oral administration of the suspension was calculated by the Loo-Riegelman method. The half-time of absorption (1.94 ± 0.92 hours) was derived from the expression:

$$t_{1/2\ (ab)} = \frac{0.693}{k_{ab}}$$ **Equation 2•2**

When the rate of absorption is much faster than that of elimination, the linear terminal phases of the semilogarithmic plots of plasma drug level–time curves after an oral (or any nonintravascular paren-

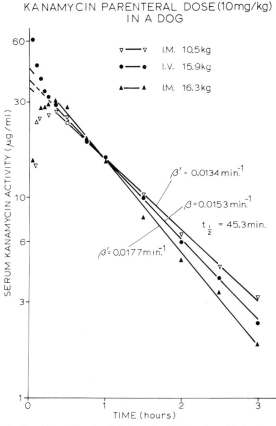

Figure 2–8 Semilogarithmic plot showing first-order elimination of kanamycin from serum of a dog after 10 mg/kg doses by the intravenous and intramuscular (on two occasions) routes.

teral route) dose and an intravenous dose are parallel, which means that their slopes are the same. The curves (plotted on semilogarithmic coordinates), depicting change in serum kanamycin activity with time in a dog after intravenous and intramuscular administration of single doses (10 mg/kg) of 5 per cent aqueous solution of kanamycin sulfate, are shown in Figure 2–8. The elimination (postabsorption and post-distribution) phases of the curves, which are represented by least squares linear regression lines based on experimental data from 20 to 180 minutes, have practically similar slopes. From the expression $t_{1/2}$ = 0.693/β (where β is the overall elimination rate constant), the half-life of kanamycin was calculated. Half-life values (mean ± S.D.) obtained in six normal beagles were 59.0 ± 8.8 min after intramuscular dosage, 57.5 ± 17.2 min after intravenous drug administration and 45.9 ± 5.7 min when dosage by the intramuscular route was repeated at a later time. Curves showing the time-related change in serum kanamycin activity after intravenous and intratracheal injection of single doses (10 mg/kg) of an aqueous solution of kanamycin sulfate

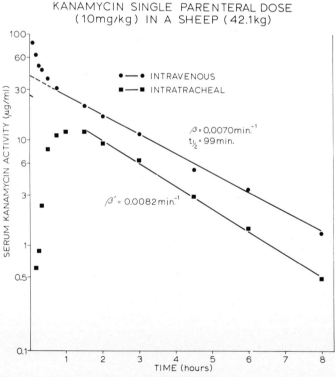

Figure 2–9 Elimination phase of curves, plotted on semilogarithmic coordinates, depicting first-order decline of serum kanamycin activity after intravenous and intratracheal administration of a fixed dose (10 mg/kg) to a sheep weighing 42.1 kg.

in a sheep are given in Figure 2–9. The linear terminal phases of the semilogarithmic curves are nearly parallel and, consequently, have similar slopes (and similar half-life values). It may be concluded that the half-life of kanamycin is independent of the route of parenteral administration. This feature is characteristic of first-order (exponential) elimination. Although rapid absorption is important, the fraction of the dose that is absorbed does not influence the rate of elimination.

The absorption rate constant for kanamycin from the intramuscular site of administration in dogs was calculated by the Loo-Riegelman method. A semilogarithmic plot showing per cent remaining to be absorbed versus time for one dog is shown in Figure 2–10. The half-time of absorption [$t_{1/2\ (ab)}$ = 9.7 min] was derived from the absorption rate constant (k_{ab}), which is the negative value of the slope of the first-order plot.

When the rate of absorption is much slower than that of elimina-

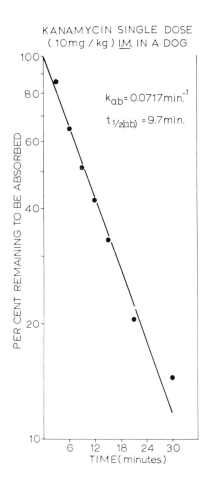

KANAMYCIN SINGLE DOSE
(10mg / kg) I.M. IN A DOG

k_{ab}= 0.0717min.$^{-1}$

$t_{1/2(ab)}$ = 9.7min.

Figure 2–10 Apparent first-order absorption of kanamycin following intramuscular administration of a single dose (10 mg/kg) to a dog. The absorption rate constant (k_{ab}) is obtained from the slope of the semilogarithmic plot of per cent drug remaining to be absorbed (unabsorbed) from injection site versus time after injection.

PER CENT REMAINING TO BE ABSORBED

TIME(minutes)

tion, absorption rather than elimination processes governs the rate of removal of the drug from the body. This situation exists for depot preparations, such as procaine penicillin G, and was found to occur with salicylate in cows given aspirin by the oral route. Because of slow absorption [$t_{1/2 \ (ab)}$ = 2.91 ± 0.37 hours] from the reticulorumen, serum salicylate concentrations declined at a much slower rate after oral dosage with aspirin (apparent elimination half-time, 3.70 ± 0.44 hours) than after intravenous administration of an equivalent dose of so-dium salicylate ($t_{1/2}$ = 0.54 ± 0.04 hours). The systemic availability of salicylate following oral administration of aspirin tablets to six normal cows was 70 per cent (Gingerich et al., 1975).

The absorption of a drug from the gastrointestinal tract is un-doubtedly a complex process. Both the rate and extent of absorption of a drug can vary quite considerably among animals. In veterinary medicine, variation among species is a most important aspect of bioavailability when the oral route of drug administration is em-ployed. Comparison of the serum level–time profiles, plotted on arith-metic coordinates, obtained after giving chloramphenicol orally (in capsules) at the same dosage rate (22 mg/kg), to ponies (8), goats (8), pigs (8), dogs (4), and cats (4) is instructive (Fig. 2–11). The max-imum concentration of chloramphenicol in serum was present at 2 or 3 hours, depending on the species. Based on the relative areas under the curves, the drug was most completely absorbed in cats. The areas under the curves would be influenced by the rate of elimination of the drug from the body, and the half-lives, obtained after intravenous dos-age, were 0.9, 2.0, 1.3, 4.2 and 5.1 hours in ponies, goats, pigs, dogs

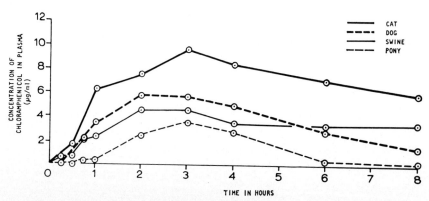

Figure 2–11 Serum concentrations of chloramphenicol in domestic animals after oral administration of chloramphenicol capsules (22 mg/kg). The drug was not detectable in serum of goats. Each point represents the mean drug concentration measured in four cats or dogs and in eight swine, ponies, or goats. (From Davis, L. E., Neff, C. A., Baggot, J. D., and Powers, T. E. [1972]: *Am. J. vet. Res.*, 33:2259–2266.)

and cats, respectively. The drug was not detected in serum of the goats, owing to reduction of the nitro group, which implies metabolic inactivation, within the ruminal environment (Theodorides et al., 1968). In a comparative study of salicylate absorption (Davis and Westfall, 1972), peak concentrations of salicylate in plasma were highest in swine and dogs and considerably lower in the herbivorous species (ponies and goats). Study of the limited data on systemic availability of orally administered drug products to domestic animals suggests that gastrointestinal absorption is fast and relatively complete in the dog, cat and pig, highly variable in the equine species and slow in ruminant animals. In carnivorous species, absorption is usually more rapid than elimination, but it may control the rate of removal and thereby prolong the action of some drugs in ruminant species. In any species, individual variations in response to a given dose of drug are more pronounced when the oral rather than parenteral route of administration is employed.

REFERENCES

Alexander, F. (1972): Certain aspects of the physiology and pharmacology of the horse's digestive tract. *Equine vet. J., 4*:166–169.

Alexanderson, B., Borgå, O. and Alván, G. (1973): The availability of orally administered nortriptyline. *Europ. J. clin. Pharmacol., 5*:181–185.

Allenby, A. C., Fletcher, J., Schock, C., and Tees, T. F. S. (1969): The effect of heat, pH and organic solvents on the electrical impedance and permeability of excised human skin. *Brit. J. Dermat. 81*(Suppl. 4): 31–39.

Annison, E. F., and Lewis, D. (1959): *Metabolism in the Rumen.* London, Methuen, p. 124.

Baggot, J. D., Ludden, T. M., and Powers, T. E. (1976): The bioavailability, disposition kinetics, and dosage of sulphadimethoxine in dogs. *Can. J. comp. Med., 40*:310–317.

Baker, H. (1968): The effects of dimethylsulfoxide, dimethylformamide, and dimethylacetamide on the cutaneous barrier to water in human skin. *J. invest. Dermat., 50*:283–288.

Barrios, S., Sorensen, J. H., and Spickett, R. G. W. (1975): Bioavailability of cephalexin after intramuscular injection of its lysine salt. *J. Pharm. Pharmacol. 27*:711–712.

Bates, T. R., and Sequeira, J. A. L. (1975): Use of 24-hr urinary excretion data to assess bioavailability of griseofulvin in humans. *J. pharm. Sci., 64*:709–710.

Bothwell, T. H. (1968): The control of iron absorption. *Brit. J. Haemat., 14*:453–456.

Bourget, L. (1893): Ueber die Resorption der Salicylsäure durch die Haut und die Behandlung des acuten gelenkrheumatismus. *Ther. Monatsh., 7*:531–539.

Boxenbaum, H. G., and Kaplan, S. A. (1975): Potential source of error in absorption rate calculations. *J. pharmacokinet. Biopharm., 3*:257–264.

Boyes, R. N., Adams, H. J., and Duce, B. R. (1970): Oral absorption and disposition kinetics of lidocaine hydrochloride in dogs. *J. Pharmacol. exp. Ther., 174*:1–8.

Brodie, B. B., and Hogben, C. A. M. (1957): Some physicochemical factors in drug action. *J. Pharm. Pharmacol., 9*:345–380.

Chiou, W. L., and Riegelman, S. (1971): Absorption characteristics of solid dispersed and micronized griseofulvin in man. *J. pharm. Sci., 60*:1376–1380.

Danielli, J. F., Hitchcock, M. W. S., Marshall, R. A., and Phillipson, A. T. (1945): The mechanism of absorption from the rumen as exemplified by the behaviour of acetic, propionic and butyric acids. *J. exp. Biol.*, *22*:75–84.

Davis, L. E., Neff, C. A., Baggot, J. D., and Powers, T. E. (1972): Pharmacokinetics of chloramphenicol in domesticated animals. *Am. J. vet. Res.*, *33*:2259–2266.

Davis, L. E., and Westfall, B. A. (1972): Species differences in biotransformation and excretion of salicylate. *Am. J. vet Res.*, *33*:1253–1262.

Dobson, A. (1967): Physiological peculiarities of the ruminant relevant to drug distribution. *Fed. Proc.*, *26*:994–1000.

Dollery, C. T., Davies, D. S., and Conolly, M. E. (1971): Differences in the metabolism of drugs, depending upon their routes of administration. *Ann. N. Y. Acad. Sci.*, *179*:108–114.

Eller, J. J., and Wolf, S. (1939): Permeability and absorptivity of skin. *Arch. Dermat. Syphilol.*, *40*:900–923.

Gamble, J. A. S., Mackay, J. S., and Dundee, J. W. (1973): Blood diazepam levels: preliminary results. *Brit. J. Anaesth.*, *45*:926–927.

Gingerich, D. A., Baggot, J. D., and Yeary, R. A. (1975): Pharmacokinetics and dosage of aspirin in cattle. *J. Am. vet. med. Assoc.*, *167*:945–948.

Gower, P. E., Dash, C. H., and O'Callaghan, C. H. (1973): Serum and blood concentration of sodium cephalexin in man given single intramuscular and intravenous injections. *J. Pharm. Pharmacol.*, *25*:376–381.

Gram, L. F., and Christiansen, J. (1975): First-pass metabolism of imipramine in man. *Clin. Pharmacol. Ther.*, *17*:555–563.

Gram, L. F., and Overø, K. F. (1975): First-pass metabolism of nortriptyline in man. *Clin. Pharmacol. Ther.*, *18*:305–314.

Gray, F. V. (1948): The absorption of volatile fatty acids from the rumen: The influence of pH on absorption. *J. exp. Biol.*, *25*:135–144.

Greenblatt, D. J., Duhme, D. W., Koch-Weser, J., and Smith, T. W. (1973): Evaluation of digoxin bioavailability in single-dose studies. *N. Engl. J. Med.*, *289*:651–654.

Greenblatt, D. J., Duhme, D. W., Koch-Weser, J., and Smith, T. W. (1974): Comparison of one- and six-day urinary digoxin excretion in single-dose bioavailability studies. *Clin. Pharmacol. Ther.*, *16*:813–816.

Hall, L. W. (1971): *Wright's Veterinary Anaesthesia and Analgesia.* 7th Ed. London, Baillière Tindall, p. 312.

Harry, R. G. (1941): Skin penetration. *Brit. J. Dermat.*, *53*:65–82.

Hogben, C. A. M., Tocco, D. J., Brodie, B. B., and Schanker, L. S. (1959): On the mechanism of the intestinal absorption of drugs. *J. Pharmacol. exp. Ther.*, *125*:275–282.

Keberle, H. (1971): Physicochemical factors of drugs affecting absorption, distribution, and excretion. *Acta Pharmacol. Toxicol.*, *29*(Suppl. 3): 30–47.

Kimura, G. (1940): Studies on absorbing coloring matter as well as heterogeneous protein through skin at time of unbalanced acid-base equilibrium; examination of skin's function of absorbing coloring matter. *Orient. J. Dis. Infants*, *28*:15.

Kligman, A. M. (1965): Topical pharmacology and toxicology of dimethyl sulfoxide. Part 1. *J.A.M.A.*, *193*:796–804.

Levy, G. (1968*a*): Dose dependent effects in pharmacokinetics. *In* D. H. Tedeschi and R. E. Tedeschi (eds.): *Importance of Fundamental Principles in Drug Evaluation.* New York, Raven Press, pp. 141–172.

Levy, G. (1968*b*): Kinetics and implications of dissolution rate limited gastrointestinal absorption of drugs. *In* E. J. Ariens (ed.): *Physicochemical Aspects of Drug Action.* Proceedings of the 3rd International Pharmacological Meeting. Vol. 7. Oxford, Pergamon Press, pp. 33–62.

Loo, J. C. K., and Riegelman, S. (1968): New method for calculating the intrinsic absorption rate of drugs. *J. pharm. Sci.*, *57*:918–928.

Lukas, G., Brindle, S. D., and Greengard, P. (1971): The route of absorption of intraperitoneally administered compounds. *J. Pharmacol. exp. Ther.*, *178*:562–566.

Masson, M. J., and Phillipson, A. T. (1951): The absorption of acetate, propionate and butyrate from the rumen of sheep. *J. Physiol.* (Lond.), *113*:189–206.

Masson, M. J., and Phillipson, A. T. (1952): The composition of the digesta leaving the abomasum of sheep. *J. Physiol.* (Lond.), *116*:98–111.

McCreesh, A. H. (1965): Percutaneous toxicity. *Toxicol. appl. Pharmacol., 7*(Suppl. 2):20–26.

Munro, D. D., and Stoughton, R. B. (1965): Dimethylacetamide (DMAC) and dimethylformamide (DMFA). Effect on percutaneous absorption. *Arch. Dermat., 92*:585–586.

Nicholas, P., Meyers, B. R., and Hirschman, S. Z. (1973): Cephalexin: Pharmacologic evalution following oral and parenteral administration. *J. clin. Pharmacol., 13*:463–468.

Phillipson, A. T., and McAnally, R. A. (1942): Studies on the fate of carbohydrates in the rumen of the sheep. *J. exp. Biol., 19*:199–214.

Riegelman, S. (1974): Pharmacokinetics: Pharmacokinetic factors affecting epidermal penetration and percutaneous absorption. *Clin. Pharmacol. Ther., 16*:873–883.

Rowland, M., Riegelman, S., and Epstein, W. L. (1968): Absorption kinetics of griseofulvin in man. *J. pharm. Sci., 57*:984–989.

Schou, J. (1961): Absorption of drugs from subcutaneous connective tissue. *Pharmacol. Rev., 13*:441–464.

Schuplein, R. J. (1965): Mechanisms of percutaneous absorption. I. Routes of penetration and influence of solubility. *J. invest. Dermat., 45*:334–346.

Schuplein, R. J., and Blank, I. H. (1971): Permeability of the skin. *Physiol. Rev., 51*:702–746.

Schwarz, C., Steinmetzer, K., and Caithaml, K. (1926): *Arch. ges. Physiol., 213*:595.

Scott, D. B., Jebson, P. J. R., Braid, D. P., Ortengren, B., and Frisch, P. (1972): Factors affecting plasma levels of lignocaine and perilocaine. *Brit. J. Anaesth., 44*:1040–1049.

Smolen, V. F. (1971): Quantitative determination of drug bioavailability and biokinetic behavior from pharmacological data for ophthalmic and oral administration of a mydriatic drug. *J. pharm. Sci., 60*:354–365.

Stoughton, R. B. (1965): Percutaneous absorption. *Toxicol. appl. Pharmacol., 7*(Suppl. 2):1–6.

Stoughton, R. B., and Fritsch, W. (1964): Influence of dimethylsulfoxide (DMSO) on human percutaneous absorption. *Arch. Dermat., 90*:512–517.

Sund, R. B., and Schou, J. (1964): The determination of absorption rates from rat muscles: an experimental approach to kinetic descriptions. *Acta Pharmacol. Toxicol. 21*:313–325.

Theodorides, V. J., DiCuollo, C. J., Guarini, J. R., and Pagano, J. F. (1968): Serum concentrations of chloramphenicol after intraruminal and intra-abomasal administration in sheep. *Am. J. Vet. Res., 29*:643–645.

Valette, G. (1953): Percutaneous absorption. *Pharm. J., 170*:461–462.

Vinson, L. J., Singer, E. J., Koehler, W. R., Lehman, M. D., and Masurat, T. (1965): The nature of the epidermal barrier and some factors influencing skin permeability. *Toxicol. appl. Pharmacol., 7*(Suppl. 2):7–19.

Wagner, J. G., and Nelson, E. (1964): Kinetic analysis of blood levels and urinary excretion in the absorptive phase after single doses of drug. *J. pharm. Sci., 53*:1392–1403.

Wilensky, A. J., and Lowden, J. A. (1973): Inadequate serum levels after intramuscular administration of diphenylhydantoin. *Neurology, 23*:318–324.

3

Drug Distribution

INTRODUCTION

Once a drug has entered the bloodstream, the concentration attained at the site of action depends upon the relative rates of the distribution and elimination processes, which proceed simultaneously. Although the blood serves as the physiological medium of translocation and exchange for all tissues, the flow of blood to various tissues differs widely (Table 3–1). Differences in regional perfusion may account for variations in the time required for drug concentrations in the tissues to equilibrate with plasma concentrations. Tissues of the central nervous system and the heart are well perfused with blood. The liver and kidneys, which are the organs responsible for elimination of the majority of drugs, constitute 2.5 per cent of the body weight and receive between 40 and 50 per cent of the cardiac output. Accessibility of drug molecules to intracellular sites of action depends upon their ability to penetrate the capillary endothelium and diffuse across the cell membrane. For drugs which do not readily cross membranes, tissue uptake may be slow or restricted, despite adequate perfusion. It is also true that moderately perfused tissues of considerable mass, such as muscle and the reticulorumen with its contents, can significantly affect the overall distribution pattern. Ruminal fluid acts as a transcellular reservoir for organic bases. Fat-soluble compounds partition slowly into the poorly perfused adipose tissue. Chronic exposure to lipophilic drugs, such as DDT or other pesticides, can cause substantial amounts to accumulate in the body fat. The adipose

48

Table 3–1   REGIONAL BLOOD FLOW IN HUMANS*

Tissue	Per Cent Body Weight	Blood Flow (ml/100 gm/min)	Per Cent Cardiac Output	
			HUMANS	DOG†
Adrenals	0.02	550	1	
Kidneys	0.4	450	24	23.1
Thyroid	0.04	400	2	
Liver: Hepatic	2	20	5	17.7
Portal		75	20	
Portal-drained viscera	2	75	20	14.3
Heart (basal)	0.4	70	4	4.9
Brain	2	55	15	
Skin	7	5	5	3.8
Muscle	40	3	15	33
Connective tissue	7	1	1	
Fat	15	1	2	

*Butler, T. C. (1962): *Proceedings of the 1st International Pharmacological Meeting.* Vol. 6. Oxford, Pergamon Press, pp. 193–212.

†Values for dogs added for comparison; data from Neff-Davis, C., Davis, L. E., and Powers, T. E. (1975): *Am. J. vet. Res., 36*:309–311.

tissue acts as a reservoir from which release is gradual, at a rate which ordinarily is too slow to provide enough circulating drug to produce observable pharmacological effects. The tetracycline antibiotics and some heavy metals persist in bone, probably by adsorption of the substances to the bone-spicule surface or incorporation into the bony lattice (Ibsen and Urist, 1964). Following absorption, inorganic lead becomes associated with erythrocytes and the soft tissues, the highest concentrations being attained in the liver and kidney. Eventually the metal is redistributed to bone, where it is deposited in the form of an insoluble salt. The fluoride ion is normally taken up in bone mineral by ion exchange (Neuman et al., 1950) and, more specifically, by exchange with hydroxyl radicals in hydroxyapatite to form fluoroapatite. To consider the translocation of fluorides to bone is therefore somewhat misleading, since the primary site of deposition of fluorides is the skeleton.

Redistribution of thiopentone into tissues less well perfused than central nervous system is responsible for the ultra-short anesthetic action of this barbiturate, produced by the rapid intravenous injection of a single small dose of the drug. If multiple doses of thiopentone are administered, however, or a continuous infusion of the drug is given, equilibrium may be attained between an anesthetic concentration in the brain and the same concentration throughout the body fluids. Under these conditions thiopentone has an extremely long duration of action, and the drug effect is terminated primarily by its sequestration in fat depots, its subsequent slow rate of metabolism, and consequent gradual lowering of the concentration in all the body tissues, including the brain.

With most drugs, only a very small proportion of the total amount in the body (absorbed dose) is at any time in direct interaction with the receptors producing the pharmacological action. Most of the drug remains in the various body fluids in solution, and a portion may be localized by binding to nonreceptor tissue components. The extent (or magnitude) of distribution largely determines the amount of drug which must be administered to produce a concentration within the therapeutic range of plasma levels.

Capillary Permeability

Tissue fluid is formed at the arterial ends of most capillaries in the body and resorbed at their venous ends. The hydrostatic pressure at the arterial end of ordinary capillaries pushes fluid and small water-soluble molecules into interstitial spaces, while the colloid (protein) osmotic pressure of blood becomes the dominant force attracting water and solutes at the venous end.

The capillaries, except those of the brain, are quite permeable to drugs, compared with cell membranes. All drug molecules of small or intermediate molecular weight (size) that are free in the circulation gain access to the extracellular interstitial spaces of most tissues in a rather short time. The degree of lipid-solubility determines the rate of diffusion of lipid-soluble molecules across the capillary endothelium, the entire surface of which is available for diffusion. Molecular size is the major determinant of transcapillary movement of water-soluble molecules, which may pass between endothelial cells. Water-soluble molecules are excluded from the extracellular fluid of the brain and the cerebrospinal fluid.

The permeability characteristics of capillaries in the kidney and the liver are related to the functions of these organs. The hydrostatic pressure, imparted to the blood by the beat of the heart, forces a "protein-poor" filtrate of plasma through the glomerular capillary membranes. Since glomerular capillaries are supplied with blood by an arteriole (afferent) and are also drained by an arteriole (efferent), they represent, as it were, a tuft of capillaries interposed in the course of an arteriole. The hydrostatic pressure is high (60 to 70 mm Hg) along their entire lengths. These capillaries function as ultrafilters and behave as if they were perforated by cylindrical pores 75 to 100 Å in diameter, occupying about 5 per cent of the capillary surface (Pappen-heimer, 1953). The remainder of the surface is water-impervious and presumably lipid in nature. In comparison, aqueous pores (about 60 Å in diameter) occupy only 0.1 per cent of the surface of muscle capillaries. The glomerular capillary wall is composed of three layers: an endothelial cell layer, a non-cellular basal lamina and an epithelial cell layer. The glomerular filtrate has in general the same composition as tissue fluid that is formed in capillaries elsewhere, which means that water and substances in simple solution pass through the capillary membrane readily, but plasma proteins are largely sieved (restrained). Albumin, which normally enters the filtrate in very low concentration, is absorbed in the proximal convoluted tubules. Since the endothelial cells which line the capillary membrane are fenestrated with pores that measure about 1000 Å (0.1 micrometer or μm) in diameter, this layer is not the semipermeable barrier of the glomerular capillary. It follows, therefore, that either the gelatinous basal lamina or the slit pores which lie between adjacent pedicels of the epithelial cells form the structural basis for the relative colloid impermeability of glomerular capillaries (Pitts, 1968). When drugs enter the liver via the hepatic portal vein, intermittent mixing with the hepatic arterial blood probably takes place before drug partitions into the sinusoids (Greenway and Stark, 1971). Fenestrae, which are generally oval in shape and have a diameter of about 1000 Å, exist as sieve plates in attenuated portions of cytoplasm that extend from the perinuclear regions of sinusoidal capillary endothelial cells (Wisse, 1970). There is no basal lamina surrounding the endothelial cells, so that molecules up to the size of the pores can enter and leave the blood passing through the liver quite readily. Thus, capillaries in the various organ systems display wide variations in their permeability to drugs.

Body Fluid Compartments

The body water, which constitutes 45 to 75 per cent of body weight, may be regarded as comprising several compartments that are functionally distinct (Fig. 3–1). The intracellular fluid is neither a continuous nor a homogeneous phase; rather, it represents the sum of the fluid contents of all the cells of the body. Somewhat more than half the total body water is contained in cells, so that intracellular water constitutes 30 to 40 per cent of body weight. The extracellular fluid includes the blood plasma (4 to 5 per cent of body weight) and the interstitial fluid (16 to 18 per cent of body weight). The distribution of fluid between the plasma and intercellular spaces is determined by the balance of the hydrostatic pressure, the colloid osmotic pressure, and the tissue-turgor pressure operative across the capillary endothelium. The whole blood volume, including the intracellular water of the

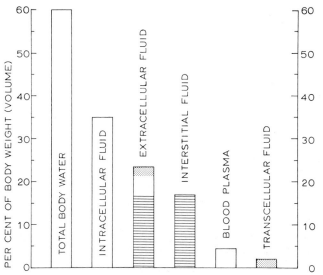

Figure 3–1 Distribution of water in the body. The relative volumes of the components of extracellular fluid are shown.

erythrocytes, accounts for 7 to 8 per cent of body weight. The transcellular fluid (1 to 3 per cent of body weight) is a specialized fraction of extracellular fluid and includes cerebrospinal, intraocular, synovial, pleural and peritoneal fluids. The common factor that distinguishes transcellular fluids from interstitial fluid is that each of the several discontinuous fractions is separated from blood plasma not only by the capillary endothelium but also by a continuous layer of epithelial cells. Although the fluid in gastrointestinal contents may be considered as extracorporeal fluid, it is important to realize that in ruminant animals the gastrointestinal contents form 12 to 15 per cent of body weight, compared with somewhat less than 1 per cent of body weight in the dog.

The total body water can be measured by determining the apparent volume of distribution of tracer water (deuterium oxide, D_2O, or tritiated water, ^3H_2O). The plasma volume is measured as the volume of distribution of a substance confined within the vascular bed, such as Evans blue, a dye of high molecular weight, or ^{131}I-serum albumin (Lombardi, 1972). In either instance, the volume of distribution of the administered substance is that of plasma albumin. It can also be estimated by measuring the volume of distribution of red blood cells tagged with radioactive phosphorus (^{32}P) or chromium (^{51}Cr). From the hematocrit, the plasma volume can be calculated. The extracellular fluid volume is less precisely determinable than is total body water or plasma volume. Many different substances (e.g., chloride and sodium ions, inulin, and radiosulfate) distribute unpredictably into the extracellular volume. Inulin tends to provide low estimates and radiosodium (^{24}Na) to provide high estimates of the volume of extracellular fluid. The volume of distribution of radiosulfate (^{35}SO$_4$) is believed to equal plasma volume plus that fraction of the interstitial volume which is in ready diffusion equilibrium with plasma; whether it is equal to the true anatomical extracellular space is unknown (Pitts, 1968). The volume of interstitial fluid is calculated as the difference between the volume of extracellular fluid and that of plasma. Intracellular water is calculated as the difference between total body water and extracellular water. The latter two calculated volumes are subject to the sum of the errors and uncertainties in measuring the component volumes.

DISTRIBUTION IN BODY FLUIDS AND TISSUES

Drug molecules in the water phase of blood plasma are available to enter the tissues of each organ at a rate determined by the blood flow to that organ, and the ability of the molecules to penetrate the capillary endothelium and diffuse into the intracellular fluid. Regional perfusion, the masses of various organs and tissues relative to body weight and the pH reaction of body fluids are the physiological parameters which determine the distribution of drugs. Certain physicochemical properties of the drug, namely, degree of lipid-solubility, extent of ionization of organic electrolytes and molecular size, together with binding affinity for plasma proteins and tissue constituents, control the distribution pattern. The dosage form and route of administration influence the bioavailability of a drug product.

There are differences in body composition among the species of domestic animals that contribute to variation in the distribution of drugs. The percentages of total body weight of various organs and tissues of dogs and goats are compared in Table 3–2. Significant species differences were observed in the contribution of several organs and tissues to the total body weights. The gastrointestinal tract and its contents constituted 4.6 per cent of the body weight of the dog compared with 20 per cent of the weight of the goat. Values for cardiac output have been reported to be 150 to 169 ml/kg/min for the dog (Sapirstein, 1958; Lombardi, 1972), and 130 ml/kg/min for the goat (Spector, 1961).

Analysis of tissues would be required for conclusive establish-

Table 3–2 PERCENTAGE OF TOTAL BODY WEIGHT OF
VARIOUS ORGANS AND TISSUES OF DOGS AND GOATS*

Organ or Tissue	Dogs ($n = 5$) Mean ± S.E.M.	Goats ($n = 8$) Mean ± S.E.M.
Muscle	54.45 ± 1.03	45.50 ± 1.10†
Skin	9.28 ± 0.57	9.24 ± 0.34
Bone	8.71 ± 1.17	6.32 ± 0.31†
Liver	2.32 ± 0.19	1.95 ± 0.17
Lungs	0.89 ± 0.06	0.88 ± 0.06
Heart	0.82 ± 0.11	0.48 ± 0.02†
Kidneys	0.61 ± 0.05	0.35 ± 0.03†
Brain	0.51 ± 0.06	0.29 ± 0.04†
Spleen	0.26 ± 0.03	0.25 ± 0.04
Gastrointestinal tract	3.87 ± 0.36	6.38 ± 0.31†
Gastrointestinal contents	0.72 ± 0.13	13.87 ± 0.74†

*Data from Neff-Davis, C., Davis, L. E., and Powers, T. E. (1975): *Am. J. vet. Res., 36*:309–311.
†Significant difference between the species (Student's *t* test, p < 0.025). S.E.M., standard error of measurement.

ment of the distribution pattern of a drug. Species variations in drug distribution frequently are based on comparison of the apparent volume of distribution (the pharmacokinetic constant). This parameter, which is derived from plasma (or serum) concentrations of the drug, provides some idea only of the extent or magnitude of distribution. A large value for the apparent volume of distribution can be interpreted to mean that the drug is widely distributed in body fluids and tissues, or that the drug is avidly bound to tissue constituents (and perhaps localized) or extensively bound to plasma proteins (if volume of distribution is derived from free drug level in plasma). A small volume of distribution could mean that the drug is restricted to certain fluid compartments of the body (e.g., extracellular fluid) or is extensively bound to plasma proteins, when volume of distribution is based on total drug concentration in plasma, or both. Most chemical assay methods measure the total (free + bound) concentration of drug in plasma. Even when protein binding is determined (e.g., by ultrafiltration or equilibrium dialysis *in vitro* at 37° C) and volume of distribution is calculated using the unbound (free) drug concentration in plasma, only tentative inferences can be made as to the anatomical distribution of the drug. Consequently, the kinetic volume of distribution reveals little about the distribution pattern of a drug. However, despite the limitation to scope of interpretation and variations due to method of computation, estimates of the magnitude of distribution provided by this kinetic parameter can be helpful in describing the disposition of drugs in the body and are essential for dosage calculations.

The high lipid-solubility of the gaseous and volatile liquid anesthetic agents enables them to enter brain extracellular fluid rapidly, but they are distributed in total body water and in most tissues. Based on their apparent volumes of distribution and measurement of tissue levels, many organic bases (e.g., amphetamine, ephedrine, quinidine, morphine) are widely distributed in body fluids and tissues (Table 3–3). Lipid-soluble bases diffuse passively into ruminal fluid, where they become trapped by ionization, so that their volumes of distribution are much larger in ruminant animals than in monogastric species (Table 3–4). The polar nature and low lipid-solubility of the aminoglycoside antibiotics (e.g., streptomycin, gentamicin, kanamycin and spectinomycin) restrict the distribution of these organic bases. Some acidic drugs (e.g., phenylbutazone, salicylates, penicillin) have small volumes of distribution (< 0.25 liter/kg), which is due to their low lipid-solubility, since they occur predominantly ionized in plasma. The sulfonamides and pentobarbitone are weak organic acids of moderate lipid-solubility, are distributed in most tissues of the body, and have volumes of distribution in the range of 0.3 to 0.8 liter/kg of body weight. The very high lipid-solubility of thiopentone enables this acidic drug to enter the various body tissues readily (Table 3–5). Whereas the intensity and duration of pharmacological activity are related to the pattern of drug distribution, there is no correlation between the rate of elimination and magnitude of distribution of drugs.

Table 3–3   DISTRIBUTION OF d-AMPHETAMINE AND QUINIDINE IN DOG TISSUES

Tissue	d-Amphetamine* (mg/kg)	Quinidine† (mg/kg)
Plasma	3.8	3.5
Cerebrospinal fluid	3.8	1.05
Liver	39.5	59.5
Lung	54.0	51.45
Spleen	35.5	79.45
Heart	14.5	—
Muscle	7.7	10.5
Brain	30.5	6.65
Kidney	68.0	63.0
Bile	3.5	16.8
Fat	1.6	—
Adrenals	—	77.0

*Axelrod, J. (1954): Studies on sympathomimetic amines. II. The biotransformation and physiological disposition of d-amphetamine, d-p-hydroxyamphetamine and d-methamphetamine. J. Pharmacol. exp. Ther., 110:315–326. © 1954 The Williams and Wilkins Company, Baltimore.

†Hiatt, E. P., and Quinn, G. P. (1945): The distribution of quinine, quinidine, cinchonine, and cinchonidine in fluids and tissues of dogs. J. Pharmacol. exp. Ther., 83:101–105. © 1945 The Williams and Wilkins Company, Baltimore.

Table 3–4 THE APPARENT SPECIFIC VOLUMES OF DISTRIBUTION (liter/kg) OF SOME DRUGS IN GOAT (OR COW), DOG, AND HORSE

Drug	Goat (Cow)	Dog	Horse
Bases:			
Amphetamine	3.08	2.67	2.61
Pentazocine	5.77	3.66	5.09
Quinidine	4.89	2.91	–
Tylosin	(1.10)	1.71	–
Chloramphenicol	1.33	1.77	1.02
Oxytetracycline	(1.04)	2.09	1.35
Kanamycin	(0.22)	0.25	0.20
Acids:			
Salicylate	(0.24)	0.19	0.18
Pentobarbitone	0.80	0.58	0.80
Sulfamethazine	(0.33)	–	0.37
Sulfadimethoxine	(0.31)	0.41	0.37
Phenylbutazone	0.26	0.18	

Although the magnitude of distribution of tetraethylammonium was unexpectedly large and significantly different (p < 0.05) in dogs (1.6 ± 0.26 liters/kg) and goats (4.0 ± 0.74 liters/kg), the rate of excretion of this compound was fast and similar ($t_{1/2} \approx 1$ hour) in both species (Neff-Davis et al., 1973). Avid binding of drugs by tissue constituents, which results in extensive localization outside the plasma, will usually retard their rate of elimination from the body. The disposition of digoxin (1 mg/100 kg body weight) in the horse provides an example of this point. The mean ($n = 5$) half-time of elimination (half-life) of digoxin was 23 hours and the apparent specific volume of distribution (corrected for plasma protein binding) was 7.3 ± 0.27 liters/kg.

Table 3–5 DISTRIBUTION OF THIOPENTONE IN VARIOUS TISSUES OF THE DOG (3.5 HOURS AFTER I.V. ADMINISTRATION OF THE DRUG)*

Tissue	Amount of Thiopentone (mg/kg)
Plasma	30.9
Plasma water	7.7
Liver	65.7
Lung	22.4
Spleen	17.4
Muscle	32.3
Heart	28.0
Fat (lumbodorsal)	136.0

*Data from Brodie, B. B., Bernstein, E., and Mark, L. C. (1952): The role of body fat in limiting the duration of action of thiopental. *J. Pharmacol. exp. Ther.*, *105*:421–426. © 1952 The Williams and Wilkins Company, Baltimore.

The extent of binding of digoxin to plasma proteins was 20 to 40 per cent at therapeutic concentrations of the drug (Francfort and Schatzmann, 1976).

The uneven distribution pattern of antimicrobial drugs in different regions of an organ can influence their efficacy in localized infections. Steady state therapeutic levels of penicillin, cephalothin, ampicillin and oxytetracycline were established in serum of dogs by giving a priming dose and then infusing each drug at a constant rate. Tissue concentrations of the antibiotics were measured in the cortical, medullary and papillary regions of the kidney (Whelton et al., 1971). The data (Table 3-6) show considerable variation in the intrarenal tissue distribution depending upon the type of antibiotic and the state of hydration of the animal. In the hydropenic state, a significant gradient of increasing concentration from cortex to papilla occurs with penicillin and cephalothin, whereas ampicillin and oxytetracycline concentrations between cortex, medulla and papilla do not differ. The increase in antibiotic concentrations from cortex to papilla was fourfold for penicillin and three-fold for cephalothin. Hydration effectively dissipated these gradients. Since the critical areas for bacterial infection in the kidney are the medullary and papillary tissues (Andriole, 1966, 1970; Beeson, 1955; Guze et al., 1961; Rocha et al., 1958), knowledge of the intrarenal distribution pattern is important in selecting antibiotics for treatment of pyelonephritis.

Blood flow rates to various parts of the brain have been estimated by measuring the rate of transfer of radioactive krypton (^{79}Kr) from blood to tissues (Kety, 1960). Several areas of the cerebral cortex have a much greater blood supply than the white matter. Auto-

Table 3-6 SERUM, TISSUE AND URINE ANTIBIOTIC CONCENTRATIONS (MEAN ± S.E.M.)*

	Serum	Cortex	Medulla	Papilla	Urine
Penicillin (units/ml)					
Hydrated	2.9 ± 0.3	12.4 ± 2.0	8.4 ± 1.2	9.3 ± 1.7	25.4 ± 2.9
Hydropenic	4.7 ± 1.1	24.9 ± 4.8	41.4 ± 4.9	99.1 ± 18.3	2478 ± 464
Cephalothin (μg/ml)					
Hydrated	15.6 ± 1.2	32.9 ± 8.0	20.8 ± 4.2	20.8 ± 3.5	91.5 ± 9.8
Hydropenic	18.2 ± 2.8	37.7 ± 7.0	52.1 ± 14	113 ± 26	3636 ± 662
Ampicillin (μg/ml)					
Hydrated	7.2 ± 0.3	56 ± 2.1	22.3 ± 2.1	20.5 ± 2.0	75.8 ± 16.8
Hydropenic	11.4 ± 0.5	42.8 ± 4.1	26.8 ± 2.0	41.8 ± 2.6	2954 ± 258
Oxytetracycline (μg/ml)					
Hydrated	1.4 ± 0.3	4.1 ± 0.6	1.9 ± 0.3	1.9 ± 0.4	3.3 ± 0.9
Hydropenic	2.4 ± 0.6	8.7 ± 0.7	6.6 ± 0.4	7.9 ± 0.8	280 ± 79

*Data from Whelton, A., Sapir, D. G., Carter, G. G., Kramer, J., and Walker, W. G. (1971): Intrarenal distribution of penicillin, cephalothin, ampicillin, and oxytetracycline during varied states of hydration. *J. Pharmacol. exp. Ther., 179*:419–428. © 1971 The Williams and Wilkins Company, Baltimore.

S.E.M., standard error of measurement.

radiographic studies have shown that certain lipophilic drugs, such as the volatile anesthetics and thiopentone, distribute initially in a manner which largely reflects the vascularization pattern. In time, the drugs become more or less uniformly distributed in the entire brain.* The distribution pattern of morphine in discrete areas of the brain did not show any specific localization of the drug (Dahlstrom and Paalzow, 1975). The plasma-to-whole brain ratio, after the intravenous administration of an analgesic dose of morphine, showed three exponential characteristics, approaching a constant value of about 4.7 to 4.8 after 4 hours. The lag time required for equilibrium between brain and plasma is a kinetic consequence of the multicompartmental characteristics of morphine.

Whole-body autoradiography is a useful technique for surveying the distribution of a drug in laboratory animals, monkeys and cats. The distribution pattern of the drug can be visually assessed in tissues and fluids that ordinarily are inaccessible by sampling techniques (Ullberg, 1954, 1963; Waddell and Brinkhous, 1967). Plasma profiles may reflect poorly the kinetic processes relevant for the pharmacological activity or for distribution of drugs with selective tissue partitioning or binding (e.g., quinacrine, chloroquine, reserpine).

Plasma Protein Binding

Drugs are transported in the circulating blood by various means. Some drugs are dissolved in plasma water, but many are partly associated with blood constituents, such as albumin, globulins, lipoproteins and erythrocytes. For the great majority of drugs, binding to plasma (or serum) albumin is quantitatively by far the most important interaction within the bloodstream. Albumin binding may influence the distribution and fate of drugs that are extensively (>80 per cent) bound. Consequently, binding may influence a drug's therapeutic efficacy, since only the unbound or free drug is available to distribute out of the vascular system and to exert pharmacological or antimicrobial activity. Once distribution equilibrium has been attained, the drug concentration in extracellular fluids will be the same as that in plasma water. It is known that only the lipid-soluble, nonionized moiety of an organic electrolyte in the water phase of blood plasma diffuses into milk and transcellular fluids (e.g., cerebrospinal and synovial). At equilibrium, the concentration of drug in the relatively protein-free transcellular fluid will approximate the free drug concentration in

---

*Roth and Barlow (1961), utilizing autoradiographic techniques, demonstrated the patterns of equilibration of a number of drugs as they entered the brain from plasma.

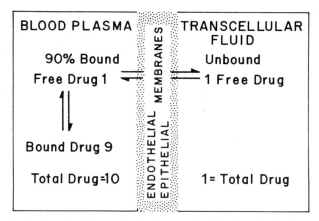

Figure 3-2 The effect of protein binding on distribution of a drug between blood plasma and transcellular fluid (relatively protein-free) — *e.g.,* cerebrospinal or synovial fluid.

plasma (Fig. 3-2). This relationship has been shown *in vivo* for cerebrospinal fluid with amphetamine (Baggot et al., 1972) and diazepam (Kanto et al., 1975), and for synovial fluid with cloxacillin and ampicillin (Howell et al., 1972). Digoxin enters milk (Rasmussen et al., 1975) and saliva (Huffman, 1975) by passive diffusion. The free drug has been shown to be in equilibrium between serum and saliva in the human. If plasma and saliva samples are obtained simultaneously, measurement of their respective drug concentrations permits one to estimate the fraction of drug bound to plasma proteins (F_b) from the plasma and salivary drug decline curves (Vesell et al., 1975):

$$F_b = 1 - \frac{(V_d)_P}{(V_d)_S} \qquad \textbf{Equation 3 • 1}$$

where $(V_d)_P$ and $(V_d)_S$ are the apparent volumes of distribution of the drug based on plasma and saliva levels, respectively. Experimental verification of Equation 3 · 1 was obtained with antipyrine, aminopyrine and phenacetin (Vesell et al., 1975), theophylline (Koysooko et al., 1974) and tolbutamide (Matin et al., 1974). For acidic drugs whose pK_a is less than 9 and for bases with pK_a greater than 5, the degree of drug ionization in plasma and saliva must be incorporated:

$$F_b = 1 - R_{P/S}\left[\frac{C^\circ_S}{C^\circ_P}\right] \qquad \textbf{Equation 3 • 2}$$

where $R_{P/S}$ is the theoretical equilibrium concentration ratio (defined in Equations 1·3 and 1·4) which takes into account plasma and salivary pH reactions as well as the pK_a value of the drug. Estimation of the extent of protein binding by this technique may be satisfactory only for drugs whose disposition kinetics can be adequately described by the one-compartment open model (see Chapter 6, *Principles of Pharmacokinetics*).

The interaction of a drug with a binding site on albumin may be considered a reversible reaction obeying the law of mass action,

$$[\text{Free drug}] + [\text{Albumin}] \underset{k_2}{\overset{k_1}{\rightleftharpoons}} [\text{Drug-Albumin Complex}] \quad \textbf{Equation 3} \cdot \textbf{3}$$

In this reaction k_1 and k_2 are the rate constants of the association and dissociation processes, respectively, and have half-times of a few milliseconds. Since the binding interaction is readily reversible, the drug-albumin complex serves as a circulating drug reservoir, which provides free drug as the concentration in plasma water declines by elimination (i.e., biotransformation and excretion) processes. At the pH of plasma (7.4), albumin has a net negative charge, but it can interact with both positive and negative charges on drugs. The electrostatic attraction of a drug molecule toward its binding site on plasma albumin is usually reinforced by hydrogen bonds, hydrophobic bonds and dipole-induced dipole bonding (Van der Waals' forces). The binding of individual drugs ranges from very little (e.g., kanamycin) to binding most of the drug in the plasma (e.g., phenylbutazone, diazepam). Slight structural modification of a molecule may significantly alter the extent of the drug-albumin interaction. While digoxin and digitoxin molecules differ only by the presence of an —OH group at the C12 position of digitoxin (Fig. 3–3), digoxin binding to plasma

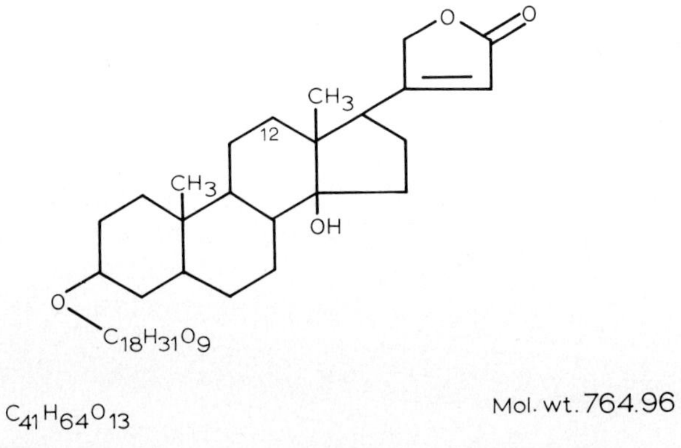

Figure 3–3 Structural formula of digitoxin. β-Hydroxylation at carbon-12 position (indicated) of the steroid nucleus produces digoxin.

proteins of the dog was 27 per cent ± 2.63 and digitoxin binding was 88.8 per cent ± 0.53 (Baggot and Davis, 1973*a*). Binding of morphine (12.1 per cent ± 0.94) and codeine (which is methylmorphine) (9.6 per cent ± 1.06) in canine plasma were in the same range (Baggot and Davis, 1973*b*).

The affinity between a drug and its binding sites is expressed as the concentration ratio of the drug in the bound form to the product of the free drug and albumin:

$$\frac{\text{[Drug-Albumin Complex]}}{\text{[Free Drug]} \times \text{[Albumin]}} = \frac{k_1}{k_2} = K_a \qquad \textbf{Equation 3 • 4}$$

where K_a is the (equilibrium) association constant, in units of liters per mole. Affinity is expressed more frequently in terms of the dissociation constant (K_d), in units of moles per liter, which is the reciprocal of the association constant (k_2/k_1) of the drug-albumin complex. The association constants (K_a) for digitoxin and digoxin binding with human serum albumin at 37°C are 9.6×10^4 liters/mole and 9.0×10^2 liters/mole, respectively (Lukas and DeMartino, 1969). Based on these values, the dissociation constants would be 1.04×10^{-5} mole/liter (M) for digitoxin and 1.11×10^{-3} mole/liter for digoxin. The total binding

Table 3–7 QUANTITATIVE ASPECTS OF DRUG–SERUM PROTEIN INTERACTION

Drug	Species	Binding Capacity (mole/g)	Dissociation Constant (molar)	Serum Protein Concentration (g/liter)	References
Penicillin G	Horse	39×10^{-6}	2.13×10^{-3}	64.0	a
Ampicillin	Horse	46.5×10^{-6}	22.7×10^{-3}	65.0	a
Digoxin	Horse	0.23×10^{-6}	35.0×10^{-6}	72.8	b
Oxytetracycline	Horse	3.9×10^{-6}	2.25×10^{-4}	64.2	c
	Cow	3.13×10^{-6}	2.15×10^{-4}	79.3	c
Chloramphenicol	Horse	9.12×10^{-6}	5.07×10^{-4}	64.2	d
	Cow	1.03×10^{-5}	8.48×10^{-4}	79.3	d
Sulfamethazine	Horse	12.99×10^{-6}	4.29×10^{-4}		e
	Cow	7.77×10^{-6}	1.35×10^{-4}		f
	Pig	10.86×10^{-6}	2.45×10^{-4}		g
Sulfadimethoxine	Horse	9.77×10^{-6}	3.61×10^{-5}		e
	Cow	9.04×10^{-6}	1.93×10^{-5}		f
	Pig	9.94×10^{-6}	3.17×10^{-5}		g

a Dürr, A. (1976): *Res. vet. Sci., 20*:24–29.
b Francfort, P., and Schatzmann, H. J. (1976): *Res. vet. Sci., 20*:84–89.
c Pilloud, M. (1973*a*): *Res. vet. Sci., 15*:224–230.
d Pilloud, M. (1973*b*): *Res. vet. Sci., 15*:231–238.
e Tschudi, P. (1972): *Zbl. vet. Med., A, 19*:851–861.
f Tschudi, P. (1973*a*): *Zbl. vet. Med., A, 20*:145–154.
g Tschudi, P. (1973*b*): *Zbl. vet. Med., A, 20*:155–165.

capacity of plasma proteins for a given drug is the product of the number of binding sites per protein molecule and the total concentration of protein. The dissociation constant of the plasma protein-drug complex (molar concentration) and the binding capacity of plasma proteins (in moles/gram of protein) are given for a number of drugs (Table 3–7). Linearization of the drug concentration data obtained from *in vitro* binding experiments (using equilibrium dialysis and ultrafiltration techniques with whole plasma) has been described by Krüger-Thiemer (1961), and Dettli and Spring (1966). The parameters were derived graphically by means of one of the plots shown in Figure 3–4. When plot *a* of Figure 3–4 is chosen, the slope of the calculated regression line yields the binding capacity of the plasma proteins for the drug, while the negative intercept

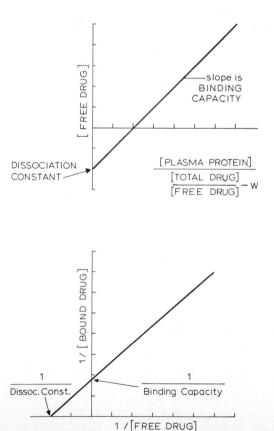

Figure 3–4 Some graphical techniques for obtaining values of parameters which describe drug interaction with plasma proteins (binding capacity and dissociation constant) from *in vitro* experiments. In upper plot, *w* is water content of serum; values of *w* for humans, dogs, and rats are 0.94, 0.93, and 0.935, respectively.

with the ordinate is equal to the dissociation constant of the drug-protein complex. Use of plot *b* becomes necessary when the dissociation constant of the drug-protein complex (moles/liter) and the total number of binding sites (i.e., binding capacity) per liter of plasma (moles/liter) are not of the same order of magnitude, as was the situation with ampicillin and digoxin. When the double reciprocal plot is employed, the dissociation constant is the negative reciprocal of the regression line intercept with the abscissa, and the total number of binding sites is the reciprocal of the intercept with the ordinate. The concentration of free drug in serum (or plasma) can be obtained from knowledge of the total drug concentration (the range of therapeutic levels is usually expressed in this form) and the parameters of binding (capacity and dissociation constant). A change in any of these variables, whether due to dosage adjustment, disease of the kidneys (uremia) or liver (hypoproteinemia), or concomitant administration of other drugs that compete for the protein binding sites will change the fraction of unbound drug. Alterations of temperature (even of $1°$ C) and pH of the solution have been shown to affect the number of binding sites and their dissociation constants *in vitro,* and these variables are encountered in the febrile state and in disturbances of acid-base balance. Although plasma protein binding can influence the distribution of drugs in the body, the magnitude of the effect depends both on the strength of association and the dosage of drug. It has been stated that only when the equilibrium association constant (K_a) exceeds 10^4 liters per mole, which corresponds to at least 83 per cent binding to plasma proteins, will changes in free drug concentration be substantial within a usual dosage range (Martin, 1965).

When a drug binds at different sites on the albumin molecule, each binding site is characterized by a distinct association constant. This means that different binding sites possess different affinities for the drug molecules. To determine the number and affinities of different binding sites, the fraction of drug bound by a solution of albumin (e.g., 6.86×10^{-4} M bovine serum albumin) is determined in phosphate buffer (0.08 molar, pH 7.4) at widely varying concentrations of free drug. A Scatchard plot (1949) of the binding data indicates the number of binding sites (n) and their association constants (K_a). This plot, on arithmetic coordinates, of r/molar concentration of free drug [D] versus r (number of moles of drug bound per mole of albumin), gives a straight line (least squares linear regression line is calculated) for each type of binding site (Fig. 3–5). The ordinate and abscissa intercepts yield nK_a and n, respectively, and the slope of the regression line gives K_a for that type of binding site. A useful feature of the Scatchard plot is that if there are distinct sets of binding sites with different affinities, two or more line segments may be dis-

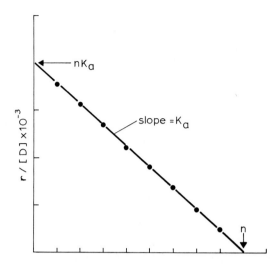

Figure 3–5 The Scatchard plot is frequently used for analysis of drug-albumin binding data. The equation may be written in the form:

$$r/[D] = nK_a - rK_a$$

where r is moles of drug bound per mole of albumin, $[D]$ represents molar concentration of free drug, n is the number of binding sites in a class per albumin molecule, and K_a is their association constant.

tinguishable. Human albumin has two classes of binding sites for furosemide ($n_1 = 1.42$, $K_{a1} = 5.07 \times 10^4$ M^{-1}; $n_2 = 3.4$, $K_{a2} = 1.58 \times 10^4$ M^{-1}); furosemide interaction with human albumin involves hydrophobic, ionic and hydrogen forces (Prandota and Pruitt, 1975). Bovine albumin has one site with a high affinity for penicillin and a large number of subsidiary sites of a very low affinity (Keen, 1966). The curvilinear appearance of the Scatchard plot of the binding of coumarin anticoagulants by human serum albumin suggests that more than one type of binding site on the albumin molecule is involved (Garten and Wosilait, 1971).

The binding of drugs to plasma proteins is usually determined by *in vitro* techniques. Statements on the fractional binding, usually expressed as "the per cent of drug bound to plasma proteins," are not very meaningful unless qualified by a statement of the drug concentration. The protein concentration and albumin fraction should also be given, as well as the state of health of the nonmedicated animals from which blood was obtained. Furthermore, all binding experiments should be performed at 37° C.

The extent of binding of various drugs to plasma proteins of dogs

Table 3–8   BINDING OF DRUGS TO PLASMA PROTEINS IN THE DOG

Drug	Concentration of Drug (μg/ml)	Extent of Binding (per cent)
Sulfadimethoxine	100	81.0
Sulfisoxazole	100	68.0
Sulfamethoxypyridazine	100	60.0
Sulfadiazine	100	17.0
Phenytoin	20	80.0
Chloramphenicol	20	39.5
Quinidine	10	75.0
Thiopentone	10	75.0
Warfarin	6.75	97.4
Morphine	1	12.1
Codeine	1	9.6
Amphetamine	0.1	27.1
Chlorpromazine	0.1	94.1
Digitoxin	0.05	88.8
Digoxin	0.01	27.0
Naltrexone	0.01	28.6

is given in Table 3–8. Drug-free blood was collected from normal dogs, and binding was measured at therapeutic concentrations of the drugs by the equilibrium dialysis technique at 37° C. Within the therapeutic range of plasma levels, the binding of most acidic drugs is inversely related to their concentration in plasma. The per cent binding of sulfonamide compounds, for example, decreases with increasing sulfonamide concentration in plasma. Protein binding of many bases (e.g., amphetamine, desmethylimipramine, morphine, naltrexone) is independent of their concentrations, but the per cent binding of some bases (e.g., methadone, quinidine, propranolol and the benzodiazepines) has been characterized as concentration dependent.

Species variations of statistical significance have been found in the degree of binding of many drugs to plasma proteins (Table 3–9). In mammalian species, however, the extent of binding of any drug is within a range which permits the binding to be classed as high (or extensive), moderately high, moderate, low and very low (or insignificant). The range of binding of different drugs to plasma proteins in the various species of domestic animals, as well as in humans, monkeys and rabbits, is presented in Table 3–10. Variation in binding does not relate to the total protein concentration in plasma, but may be attributed, at least tentatively, to differences in the composition and conformation of plasma albumins. The total protein and albumin concentrations of chicken plasma are about half those in mammalian species, and binding of drugs to plasma proteins in chickens is proportionately lower. It is interesting to note that ovalbumin shows little af-

Table 3–9 EXTENT OF BINDING OF DRUGS TO PLASMA (OR SERUM) PROTEINS AT THERAPEUTIC CONCENTRATIONS

Drug	Concentration (μg/ml)	Percentage Bound				References
		HUMAN	RUMINANT	ANIMAL	DOG	
Salicylate	200	85	62	Goat	60	Davis, L. E., and Westfall, B. A. (1972): *Am. J. vet. Res.,* 33:1253–1262.
Sulfadiazine	100	33	24	Cow	17	Anton, A. H. (1960): *J. Pharmacol. exp. Ther.,* 129:282–290.
Sulfisoxazole	100	84	76	Cow	68	Anton, A. H. (1960): *J. Pharmacol. exp. Ther.,* 129:282–290.
Sulfadimethoxine	100	–	83	Cow	81	
Chloramphenicol	20	46	30	Goat	39.5	Davis, L. E., et al. (1972): *Am. J. vet. Res.,* 33:2259–2266.
Cloxacillin	20	95.2[a]	71.3	Cow[b]	64.5[c]	
Benzylpenicillin	10	64.6[a]	48.3	Cow[d]	–	
Phenytoin	10	87	82.5	Cow	81	Baggot, J. D., and Davis, L. E. (1973c): *Comp. gen. Pharmacol.,* 4:399–404.
Lincomycin	5	72[e]	34.2	Ewe[b]	–	
Kanamycin	5	2.8[f]	4.0	Ewe[b]	–	
Morphine	1	34[g]	23.6	Cow	12.1	Baggot, J. D., and Davis, L. E. (1973b): *Am. J. vet. Res.,* 34:571–574
Digitoxin	0.05	92.3	86.6	Cow	88.8	Baggot, J. D., and Davis, L. E. (1973a): *Res. vet. Sci.,* 15:81–87.

[a]Kunin, C. M. (1967): *Ann. N. Y. Acad. Sci., 145*:282–290.
[b]Ziv, G., and Sulman, F. G. (1972): *Antimicrob. Agents Chemother., 2*:206–213.
[c]Acred, P., et al., (1970): *Brit. J. Pharmacol., 39*:439–446.
[d]Keen, P. M. (1965): *Brit. J. Pharmacol., 25*:507–514.
[e]Gordon, R. C., et al. (1973): *J. Pharmacol. Sci., 62*:1074–1077.
[f]Gordon, R. C., et al. (1972): *Antimicrob. Agents Chemother., 2*:214–216.
[g]Olsen, G. D. (1975): *Clin. Pharmacol. Ther., 17*:31–35.

finity for drugs that are bound appreciably to serum albumins. While no pattern of drug-protein binding is discernible, humans appear to bind acidic drugs more extensively than do domestic animals. Species variations in plasma protein binding of a drug will contribute to differences in the disposition of the drug only when the binding is extensive. The apparent volume of distribution (based on total drug con-

Table 3–10 RANGE OF DRUG BINDING TO PLASMA PROTEINS OF MAMMALIAN SPECIES AT THERAPEUTIC CONCENTRATIONS*

Drug	Range of Binding (per cent)
Digitoxin	83 to 93
Phenytoin	73 to 85
Sulfisoxazole	65 to 86
Amphetamine	20 to 40
Digoxin	18 to 36
Morphine	12 to 20
Codeine	7 to 16

*Total protein concentration in plasma of all the mammalian species is within the range 6.0 to 8.5 g per 100 ml.

centration in plasma) can be misleadingly small. For such drugs (e.g., phenylbutazone, phenytoin), it would be more informative to calculate volume of distribution on the basis of free drug concentration in plasma. To fully appreciate the significance of plasma protein binding, the fraction bound in plasma must be considered in conjunction with the overall magnitude of distribution of the drug in the tissues. Even though binding to plasma proteins may be extensive, only a small fraction of the total dose is present in the plasma when the drug is widely distributed in the tissues. This is the situation with some lipophilic organic bases (e.g., diazepam, quinidine). The situation is quite different with acidic drugs, such as phenylbutazone and warfarin, in which a significant fraction of the total dose is present in the plasma. A significant increase in the unbound fraction of an acidic drug in plasma, whether it results from competitive displacement by another drug from albumin binding sites or from the presence of uremia, will cause enhanced pharmacological activity. Drugs or drug metabolites are most likely to displace other drugs from albumin binding sites if they have a high affinity for albumin and are present in high concentrations in plasma during therapy (e.g., phenylbutazone and oxyphenbutazone). The concomitant administration of phenylbutazone and warfarin to dogs resulted in an elevation of the free fraction of warfarin in the plasma from 2.6 to 8.0 per cent, owing to decreased binding of warfarin to plasma proteins. The potentiated anticoagulant response (hypoprothrombinemia) to warfarin associated with phenylbutazone administration was accompanied by a two-fold decrease in the plasma half-life of warfarin (from 18.4 hours in control animals to 9.6 hours in phenylbutazone-treated dogs), displacement from binding sites making the drug more readily available for metabolism and excretion (Bachmann and Burkman, 1975). The extent of albumin binding of phenytoin, pentobarbitone and the cardiac glycosides (digitoxin and digoxin) is decreased in the presence of uremia—i.e., in animals with impaired renal function. Consequences of the decreased protein binding include a lower fraction of the dose in the uremic plasma, a higher apparent volume of distribution, and an enhanced pharmacological effect. The overall elimination rate constant for phenytoin was greater (shorter half-life) in uremic patients than in normal humans (Odar-Cederlöf and Borgå, 1974). However, this difference might be due mainly to induction of phenytoin metabolism in the uremic state. Although pentobarbitone can be safely used to anesthetize dogs with impaired renal function (Davis et al., 1973), it is important to bear in mind that the uremic animal may show an increased sensitivity to action of the barbiturate (Richards et al., 1953).

Since albumin does not pass through the glomerular membrane to an appreciable extent, the albumin-bound drug is not filtered in the renal glomerulus. Consequently, binding to plasma albumin delays the excretion of drugs by reducing their availability for glomerular filtration. The slow elimination of sulfadimethoxine ($t_{1/2}$ = 12.5 hours in the cow, 13.2 hours in the dog) is mainly due to extensive binding of this sulfonamide to plasma albumin. Protein binding does not retard carrier-mediated transport processes, such as renal tubular excretion of penicillins and furosemide. The drug-albumin interaction is so rapidly reversible that free drug molecules withdrawn from the blood plasma by a specialized transport process are replaced instantly by free drug derived from dissociation of the drug-albumin complex. Although cloxacillin and ampicillin have the same half-life in the cow (1.2 hours), cloxacillin is about 75 per cent bound while ampicillin is only 18 per cent bound to serum albumin. The half-lives of benzylpenicillin and phenoxymethylpenicillin in the cow are also the same (0.7 hour), but their extent of binding to serum albumin is 50 per cent and 65 per cent, respectively. Even though the fate of penicillin analogues is similar, their binding to serum albumin differs markedly in any species and does not correlate with their rate of elimination. Binding does, however, influence the serum and tissue levels obtained after administration of any given dose. The greater the degree of binding, the higher the total penicillin concentration in the serum, only a fraction of which, however, is diffusible and active (bactericidal).

The fate of drug molecules which have entered the hepatocyte determines the influence of binding to plasma proteins on hepatic handling of the drugs. Since only free drug molecules in the plasma can diffuse into the hepatocyte, albumin binding decreases the availability of drug at any time to the site of biotransformation. The hepatic metabolism, principally acetylation, of certain sulfonamide compounds was shown to be inversely related to their extent of albumin binding (Wiseman and Nelson, 1964). Extensive binding to plasma albumin will restrict somewhat the distribution of lipophilic bases so that binding will increase their availability to hepatocytes, with their microsomal drug-metabolizing enzymes. The rapid hepatic extraction of propranolol is the result of high-affinity drug uptake into the liver (probably due to tissue binding), a process that is dose-dependent (Evans et al., 1973). The limited extravascular distribution will also increase the overall rate of elimination of drugs which are excreted in bile (unchanged or as conjugates) by a carrier-mediated transport process. Propranolol and bromsulfthalein are highly bound to plasma albumin and have high hepatic clearance values. It may be concluded that the influence of extensive (> 80 per cent) binding to plasma proteins on the rate of drug elimination depends on the efficiency of the elimination (biotransformation and excretion) processes. Moderate and low extents of protein binding have relatively little influence on the distribution and elimination of drugs, since the drug-albumin interaction is readily reversible.

Distribution in Whole Blood

The binding of drugs to erythrocytes and other cellular components of blood has received little attention. Drugs are known to penetrate the erythrocyte at a rate that is roughly related to their lipid-to-water partition coefficient (Schanker et al., 1964). Pentazocine, which is highly lipid-soluble, rapidly attained equilibrium between blood cells and plasma (Ehrnebo et al., 1974). In normal human subjects, 48 per cent of the total amount of pentazocine in whole blood is present in blood cells and 33 per cent is bound to plasma proteins; the remaining 19 per cent is in the plasma water. Abshagen and colleagues (1971) reported that 6.8 per cent of the total blood digitoxin concentration is erythrocyte bound. Human blood cells bind "appreciable proportions" of salicylate and phenobarbital (McArthur et al., 1971). Chlorthalidone and acetazolamide are both inhibitors of carbonic anhydrase, the latter being the more potent (Pulver et al., 1962). These drugs are transported in the blood partly within erythrocytes. They use and compete for the same binding sites (probably carbonic anhydrase) in the blood cells, with the affinity for acetazolamide being greater (Beermann et al., 1975). Acetazolamide is able not only to inhibit the uptake of chlorthalidone into the red cells but also to displace chlorthalidone already attached to the binding sites. Studies on the distribution of a drug in the circulating blood should, therefore, include measurements of binding to blood cells as well as to plasma proteins.

REFERENCES

Abshagen, U., Kewitz, H., and Rietbrock, N. (1971): Distribution of digoxin, digitoxin and ouabain between plasma and erythrocytes in various species. *Arch. Pharmacol., 270*:105–116.

Acred, P., Brown, D. M., Clark, B. F., and Mizen, L. (1970): The distribution of antibacterial agents between plasma and lymph in the dog. *Brit. J. Pharmacol., 39*:439–446.

Andriole, V. T. (1966): Acceleration of the inflammatory response of the renal medulla by water diuresis. *J. clin. Invest., 45*:847–854.

Andriole, V. T. (1970): Water, acidosis, and experimental pyelonephritis. *J. clin. Invest., 49*:21–30.

Anton, A. H. (1960): The relation between the binding of sulfonamides to albumin and their antibacterial efficacy. *J. Pharmacol. exp. Ther., 129*:282–290.

Axelrod, J. (1954): Studies on sympathomimetic amines. II. The biotransformation and physiological disposition of *d*-amphetamine, *d*-p-hydroxyamphetamine and *d*-methamphetamine. *J. Pharmacol. exp. Ther., 110*:315–326.

Bachmann, K. A., and Burkman, A. M. (1975): Phenylbutazone-warfarin interaction in the dog. *J. Pharm. Pharmacol., 27*:832–836.

Baggot, J. D., and Davis, L. E. (1973a): Plasma protein binding of digitoxin and digoxin in several mammalian species. *Res. vet. Sci., 15*:81–87.

Baggot, J. D., and Davis, L. E. (1973b): Species differences in plasma protein binding of morphine and codeine. *Am. J. vet. Res., 34*:571–574.

Baggot, J. D., and Davis, L. E. (1973c): Comparative study of plasma protein binding of diphenylhydantoin. *Comp. gen. Pharmacol., 4*:399–404.

Baggot, J. D., Davis, L. E., and Neff, C. A. (1972): Extent of plasma protein binding of amphetamine in different species. *Biochem. Pharmacol., 21*:1813–1816.

Beeson, P. B. (1955): Factors in the pathogenesis of pyelonephritis. *Yale J. Biol. Med., 28*:81–104.

Beermann, B., Hellstrom, K., Lindstrom, B., and Rosen, A. (1975): Binding-site interaction of chlorthalidone and acetazolamide, two drugs transported by red blood cells. *Clin. Pharmacol. Ther., 17*:424–432.

Brodie, B. B., Bernstein, E., and Mark, L. C. (1952): The role of body fat in limiting the duration of action of thiopental. *J. Pharmacol. exp. Ther., 105*:421–426.

Butler, T. C. (1962): Duration of action of drugs as affected by tissue distribution. *In* B. B. Brodie and E. G. Erdös (eds.): *Metabolic Factors Controlling Duration of Drug Action.* Proceedings of the 1st International Pharmacological Meeting, Vol. 6. Oxford, Pergamon Press, pp. 193–212.

Dahlstrom, B. E., and Paalzow, L. K. (1975): Pharmacokinetics of morphine in plasma and discrete areas of the rat brain. *J. pharmacokin. Biopharm., 3*:293–302.

Davis, L. E., Baggot, J. D., Neff-Davis, C. A., and Powers, T. E. (1973): Elimination kinetics of pentobarbital in nephrectomized dogs. *Am. J. vet. Res., 34*:231–233.

Davis, L. E., Neff-Davis, C. A., Baggot, J. D., and Powers, T. E. (1972): Pharmacokinetics of chloramphenicol in domesticated animals. *Am. J. vet Res., 33*:2259–2266.

Davis, L. E., and Westfall, B. A. (1972): Species differences in biotransformation and excretion of salicylate. *Am. J. vet. Res., 33*:1253–1262.

Dettli, L., and Spring, P. (1966): Pharmakokinetik der chemotherapeutika: theorie und praxis. *Regensb. Jb. ärztl. Fortbildung, B, 14*:17–26.

Dürr, A. (1976): Comparison of the pharmacokinetics of penicillin G and ampicillin in the horse. *Res. vet. Sci., 20*:24–29.

Ehrnebo, M., Agurell, S., Boréus, L. O., Gordon, E., and Lönroth, U. (1974): Pentazocine binding to blood cells and plasma proteins. *Clin. Pharmacol. Ther., 16*:424–429.

Evans, G. H., Wilkinson, G. R., and Shand, D. G. (1973): The disposition of propranolol. IV. A dominant role for tissue uptake in the dose-dependent extraction of propranolol by the perfused rat liver. *J. Pharmacol. exp. Ther., 186*:447–454.

Francfort, P., and Schatzmann, H. J. (1976): Pharmacological experiments as a basis for the administration of digoxin in the horse. *Res. vet. Sci., 20*:84–89.

Garten, S., and Wosilait, W. D. (1971): Comparative study of the binding of coumarin anticoagulants and serum albumins. *Biochem. Pharmacol., 20*:1661–1668.

Gordon, R. C., Regamey, C., and Kirby, W. M. M. (1972): Serum protein binding of the aminoglycoside antibiotics. *Antimicrob. Agents Chemother., 2*:214–216.

Gordon, R. C., Regamey, C., and Kirby, W. M. M. (1973): Serum protein binding of erythromycin, lincomycin, and clindamycin. *J. pharm. Sci., 62*:1074–1077.

Greenway, C. V., and Stark, R. D. (1971): Hepatic vascular bed. *Physiol. Rev., 51*:23–64.

Guze, L. B., Goldner, B. H., and Kalmanson, G. M. (1961): Pyelonephritis. I. Observations on the course of chronic non-obstructed enterococcal infection in the kidney of the rat. *Yale J. Biol. Med., 33*:372–385.

Hiatt, E. P., and Quinn, G. P. (1945): The distribution of quinine, quinidine, cinchonine and cinchonidine in fluids and tissues of dogs. *J. Pharmacol. exp., Ther., 83*:101–105.

Howell, A., Sutherland, R., and Rolinson, G. N. (1972): Effect of protein binding on levels of ampicillin and cloxacillin in synovial fluid. *Clin. Pharmacol. Ther., 13*:724–732.

DRUG DISTRIBUTION 71

Huffman, D. H. (1975): Relationship between digoxin concentrations in serum and saliva. *Clin. Pharmacol. Ther.*, *17*:310–312.

Ibsen, K. H., and Urist, M. R. (1964): The biochemistry and physiology of the tetracyclines. *Clin. Orthop.*, *32*:142–169.

Kanto, J., Kangas, L., and Siirtola, T. (1975): Cerebrospinal-fluid concentrations of diazepam and its metabolites in man. *Acta Pharmacol. Toxicol.*, *36*:328–334.

Keen, P. M. (1965): The binding of three penicillins in the plasma of several mammalian species as studied by ultrafiltration at body temperature. *Brit. J. Pharmacol.*, *25*:507–514.

Keen, P. M. (1966): The binding of penicillins to bovine serum albumin. *Biochem. Pharmacol.*, *15*:447–463.

Kety, S. S. (1960): The cerebral circulation In J. Field, H. W. Magoun, and V. E. Hall (eds.): *Handbook of Physiology*, Vol. III. Washington, D.C., American Physiological Society.

Koysooko, R., Ellis, E. F., and Levy, G. (1974): Relationship between theophylline concentration in plasma and saliva of man. *Clin. Pharmacol. Ther.*, *15*:454–460.

Krüger-Thiemer, E. (1961): Theorie der wirkung bakteriostatischer chemotherapeutika. *Jahresbericht Borstel, B*, *5*:316–400.

Kunin, C. M. (1967): Clinical significance of protein binding of the penicillins. *Ann. N.Y. Acad. Sci.*, *145*:282–290.

Lombardi, M. H. (1972): Radioisotopic blood volume and cardiac output in dogs. *Am. J. vet. Res.*, *33*:1825–1834.

Lukas, D. S., and DeMartino, A. G. (1969): Binding of digitoxin and some related cardenolides to human plasma proteins. *J. clin. Invest.*, *48*:1041–1053.

Martin, B. K. (1965): Potential effect of the plasma proteins on drug distribution. *Nature* (London), *207*:274–276.

Matin, S. B., Wan, S. H., and Karam, J. H. (1974): Pharmacokinetics of tolbutamide: Prediction by concentration in saliva. *Clin. Pharmacol. Ther.*, *16*:1052–1058.

McArthur, J. N., Dawkins, P. O., and Smith, M. J. H. (1971): The binding of indomethacin, salicylate and phenobarbitone to human whole blood *in vitro*. *J. Pharm. Pharmacol.*, *23*:32–36.

Neff-Davis, C. A., Davis, L. E., and Baggot, J. D. (1973): Pharmacokinetics of tetraethylammonium in cats, dogs, and goats. *Am. J. vet. Res.*, *34*:425–426.

Neff-Davis, C., Davis, L. E., and Powers, T. E. (1975): Comparative body compositions of the dog and goat. *Am. J. vet. Res.*, *36*:309–311.

Neuman, W. F., Neuman, M. W., Main, E. R., O'Leary, J., and Smith, F. A. (1950): The surface chemistry of bone. II. Fluoride deposition. *J. Biol. Chem.*, *187*:655–661.

Odar-Cederlöf, I., and Borgå, O. (1974): Kinetics of diphenylhydantoin in uraemic patients: consequences of decreased plasma protein binding. *Europ. J. clin. Pharmacol.*, *7*:31–37.

Olsen, G. D. (1975): Morphine binding to human plasma proteins. *Clin. Pharmacol. Ther.*, *17*:31–35.

Pappenheimer, J. R. (1953): Passage of molecules through capillary walls. *Physiol. Rev.*, *33*:387–423.

Pilloud, M. (1973*a*): Pharmacokinetics, plasma protein binding and dosage of oxytetracycline in cattle and horses. *Res. vet. Sci.*, *15*:224–230.

Pilloud, M. (1973*b*): Pharmacokinetics, plasma protein binding and dosage of chloramphenicol in cattle and horses. *Res. vet. Sci.*, *15*:231–238.

Pitts, R. F. (1968): *Physiology of the Kidney and Body Fluids*. 2nd Ed. Chicago, Year Book Medical Publishers, pp. 22–43, 54–61.

Prandota, J., and Pruitt, A. W. (1975): Furosemide binding to human albumin and plasma of nephrotic children. *Clin. Pharmacol. Ther.*, *17*:159–166.

Pulver, E., Stenger, E. G., and Exer, B. (1962): Über die hemmung der carboanhydrase durch saluretica. Naunyn-Schmiedebergs Arch. Pharmacol., *244*:195–210.

Rasmussen, F., Nawaz, M., and Steiness, E. (1975): Mammary excretion of digoxin in goats. *Acta Pharmacol. Toxicol.*, *36*:377–381.

Richards, R. K., Taylor, J. D., and Kueter, K. E. (1953): Effect of nephrectomy on the duration of sleep following administration of thiopental and hexobarbital. *J. Pharmacol. exp. Ther.*, *108*:461–473.

Rocha, H., Guze, L. B., Freedman, L. R., and Beeson, P. B. (1958): Experimental pyelonephritis. III. The influence of localized injury in different parts of the kidney on susceptibility to bacillary infection. *Yale J. Biol. Med., 30*:341–354.

Roth, L. J., and Barlow, C. F. (1961): Drugs in the brain. *Science, 134*:22–31.

Sapirstein, L. A. (1958): Regional blood flow by fractional distribution of indicators. *Am. J. Physiol., 193*:161–168.

Scatchard, G. (1949): The attractions of proteins for small molecules and ions. *Ann. N.Y. Acad. Sci., 51*:660–692.

Schanker, L. S., Johnson, J. M., and Jeffrey, J. J. (1964): Rapid passage of organic anions into human red cells. *Am. J. Physiol., 207*:503–508.

Spector, W. S. (ed.) (1961): *Handbook of Biological Data.* Philadelphia, W. B. Saunders Co.

Tschudi, P. (1972): Elimination, plasmaproteinbindung und dosierung einiger sulfonamide. I. Pferd, *Zbl. vet. Med., A, 19*:851–861.

Tschudi, P. (1973a): Elimination, plasmaproteinbindung und dosierung einiger sulfonamide. II. Untersuchungen beim rind. *Zbl. vet. Med., A., 20*:145–154.

Tschudi, P. (1973b): Elimination, plasmaproteinbindung und dosierung einiger sulfonamide. III. Untersuchungen beim schwein. *Zbl. vet. Med., A, 20*:155–165.

Ullberg, S. (1954): Studies on the distribution and fate of ^{35}S-labelled benzylpenicillin in the body. *Acta Radiol.* (Stockholm), Suppl. *118*:1–110.

Ullberg, S. (1963): Autoradiographic localization in the tissues of drugs and metabolites. *In* O. H. Lowry and P. Lindgren (eds.): *Methods for the Study of Pharmacological Effects at Cellular and Subcellular Levels.* Proceedings of the 1st International Pharmacological Meeting, Vol. 5, Oxford, Pergamon Press, pp. 29–38.

Vesell, E. S., Passananti, G. T., Glenwright, P. A., and Dvorchik, B. H. (1975): Studies on the disposition of antipyrine, aminopyrine, and phenacetin using plasma, saliva, and urine. *Clin. Pharmacol. Ther., 18*:259–272.

Waddell, W. J., and Brinkhous, W. K. (1967): The Ullberg technique of whole body autoradiography. *J. Biol. photographic Assc., 35*:147–154.

Whelton, A., Sapir, D. G., Carter, G. G., Kramer, J., and Walker, W. G. (1971): Intrarenal distribution of penicillin, cephalothin, ampicillin and oxytetracycline during varied states of hydration. *J. Pharmacol. exp. Ther., 179*:419–428.

Wiseman, E. H., and Nelson, E. (1964): Correlation of *in vivo* metabolism rate and physical properties of sulfonamides. *J. pharm. Sci., 53*:992.

Wisse, E. (1970): An electron microscopic study of the fenestrated endothelial lining of rat liver sinusoids. *J. Ultrastructur. Res., 31*:125–150.

Ziv, G., and Sulman, F. G. (1972): Binding of antibiotics to bovine and ovine serum. *Antimicrob. Agents Chemother., 2*:206–213.

4

Comparative Patterns of Drug Biotransformation

INTRODUCTION

Several factors influence the plasma (or serum) concentrations of a drug obtainable after administration of a given dose. The route of administration and bioavailability of the dosage form, the extent of binding to plasma proteins and the magnitude of extravascular distribution determine the range of plasma concentrations during the initial phase. After distribution equilibrium has been reached, the sole factor controlling the decline of drug concentration in plasma is the rate of elimination. Metabolism in the liver and renal excretion are the principal mechanisms for elimination of the majority of drugs. The efficiency of the process is frequently determined by the accessibility of drug to the sites of elimination. Consequently, the magnitude of the dosage and pattern of distribution can control the persistence of a drug in the body. Avid binding to tissue constituents or deposition in the substance of a tissue protects that fraction of the dose from elimination. In addition, the poor blood supply to adipose tissue delays the complete removal of highly lipophilic drugs from the body. Species variations in absorption, distribution and elimination processes complicate the uptake, disposition, activity and fate of drugs.

73

PATHWAYS OF BIOTRANSFORMATION

Drugs undergo biotransformation to products that are more polar and less lipid-soluble, and these metabolites have diminished activity or are inactive. The enzymes that catalyze drug transformations are found mainly in the liver, although they are also present in lesser amounts in other tissues, such as intestine, kidney, lung and blood plasma. Some metabolic reactions of drugs are carried out by the gut microflora, and certain drugs undergo spontaneous reactions under

Table 4–1   EFFECT OF PHASE I METABOLIC REACTIONS ON PHARMACOLOGICAL ACTIVITY OF DRUGS

Drug	Metabolite
Conversion of active drug to inactive metabolite	
Pentobarbital	Pentobarbital alcohol
Phenobarbital	*p*-Hydroxyphenobarbital
Phenytoin	*p*-Hydroxyphenyl derivative
Amphetamine	*p*-Hydroxyamphetamine, phenylacetone
Methylphenidate	Ritalinic acid
Meperidine	Meperidinic acid
Phenothiazine	Phenothiazine sulfoxide
Lidocaine	3-Hydroxylidocaine, 4-hydroxy-2,6-dimethylaniline
Procaine	*p*-Aminobenzoic acid
Chloramphenicol	"Arylamine"
Griseofulvin	6-Demethylgriseofulvin
Conversion of active drug to metabolite with different activity	
Propranolol	4-Hydroxypropranolol
Lidocaine	Monoethylglycinexylidide
Digitoxin	Digoxin
Phenylbutazone	Oxyphenbutazone
Phenacetin	Acetaminophen
Methamphetamine	Amphetamine
Codeine	Morphine
Meperidine	Normeperidine
Diazepam	N-Desmethyldiazepam
Imipramine	Desipramine
Primidone	Phenobarbital, phenylethylmalonamide
Acetylsalicylic acid	Salicylic acid
*Transformation of inactive drug (pro-drug) into active metabolite**	
Chloral hydrate	Trichloroethanol
Parathion	Paraoxon
Prontosil	Sulfanilamide
L-Dopa	Dopamine
Hetacillin	Ampicillin
Cephalothin	Desacetylcephalothin

*Pro-drugs, which include latentiated drug derivatives, are compounds which undergo biotransformation prior to exhibiting their pharmacological effects.

appropriate physical conditions, such as pH. The site of drug transformations may make certain routes of administration unsuitable for therapy.

The metabolic reactions which drugs undergo can be classified as oxidations, reductions, hydrolyses and syntheses (or conjugation). Because of the nature of these reactions and the biological activity of the products, it is convenient to regard the metabolism of drugs as generally occurring in two phases (Williams, 1959). The oxidations, reductions and hydrolyses occur in the first phase and can result in the inactivation of the drug, the conversion of an active drug into an active metabolite (which may act as a drug in its own right) or the activation of an initially inactive drug (Table 4-1).* The second phase of drug metabolism consists of synthetic reactions with endogenous substances (such as acetate, glycine, sulfate or glucuronic acid); the conjugated products are water-soluble and invariably are inactive. This concept of drug metabolism can be represented as in Figure 4-1. The general pattern of drug metabolism is the same in all species of animals, but wide variations in the amounts of metabolites formed are usual among species. Biotransformation frequently involves several competing pathways simultaneously, and the amounts of the metabolites formed depend on the relative rates of the various metabolic reactions. Phase I reactions usually introduce into the drug molecule groups such as OH, COOH and NH_2, which enable the phase I products to undergo the synthetic reactions. If the drug already contains a suitable chemical group, it can undergo conjugation directly, without

---

*Drug latentiation is defined as the chemical modification of a biologically active compound to form a derivative which upon *in vivo* enzymatic attack will liberate the parent drug. Examples include the acetonide derivatives of triamcinolone and fluocinolone, which improve percutaneous absorption of the steroids.

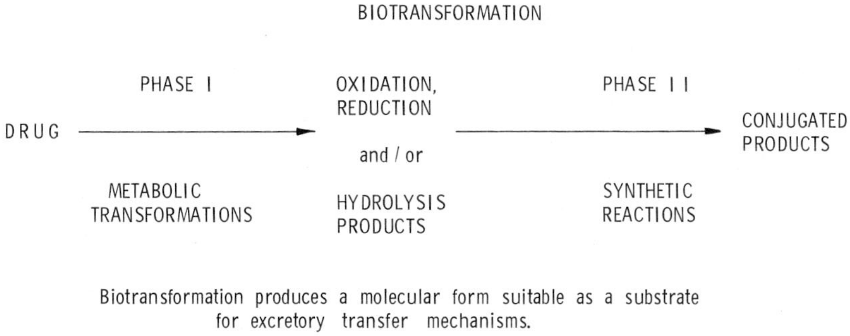

BIOTRANSFORMATION

	PHASE I	OXIDATION, REDUCTION	PHASE I I	
DRUG	——————————————→	and / or	——————————————→	CONJUGATED PRODUCTS
	METABOLIC TRANSFORMATIONS	HYDROLYSIS PRODUCTS	SYNTHETIC REACTIONS	

Biotransformation produces a molecular form suitable as a substrate
for excretory transfer mechanisms.

Figure 4–1 General pattern of drug metabolism. (After Williams, R. T. [1967]:
Fed. Proc., 26:1029–1039).

the intervention of a phase I reaction. Biotransformation tends to yield less lipid-soluble, polar compounds, which are readily excreted. Decreased lipid-solubility of a drug metabolite does not necessarily mean increased water-solubility. The antibacterial sulfonamides, for example, are metabolized to more polar, less lipid-soluble acetyl derivatives, but some of these (e.g., acetylsulfathiazole) are less water-soluble than their parent compounds. While most metabolic reactions are first-order reactions at the usual concentrations of drug obtained after administration of therapeutic doses, some metabolic pathways have a limited capacity (i.e., obey zero-order kinetics) above a certain concentration of substrate. An important consequence of a limited-capacity elimination process is that the removal of the drug from the body is disproportionately prolonged with increasing dose. As a consequence, when such drugs are used in a multiple dose regimen, the potential for excessive accumulation and toxicity is far greater.

Phase I Metabolic Reactions

The phase I metabolic reactions of drugs are carried out by enzymes that are located predominantly in the liver, although some metabolizing activity is present also in certain extrahepatic tissues, such as the kidney and intestinal mucosa and, to a lesser extent, the lungs and blood plasma. The oxidative metabolism of many drugs and steroid hormones, as well as other phase I metabolic reactions and glucuronide conjugation, is mediated by microsomal enzymes, which are associated with the so-called "smooth-surfaced" endoplasmic reticulum of hepatic cells (Fouts, 1961). A diagram of a typical hepatic parenchymal cell (hepatocyte) is shown in Figure 4–2. On homogenization of the liver, the endoplasmic reticulum is disrupted, giving rise to small vesicles, which can be separated from the homogenate by high-speed centrifugation, yielding the fraction called microsomes. Enzymes of the microsomal fraction can catalyze metabolic reactions only of compounds which are lipid-soluble at physiological pH.

Microsomal oxidation is the most general and prominent metabolic pathway for lipid-soluble drugs in mammalian species. The microsomal oxidizing enzymes have a specific requirement for reduced nicotinamide adenine dinucleotide phosphate (NADPH) and molecular oxygen (O_2), and have been classified as mixed-function oxidases (Mason, 1957). It has been shown that the microsomal hydroxylating system contains at least two catalytic components: a cytochrome called P-450 (Omura and Sato, 1964a, b), and the flavoprotein catalyzing the reduction of this cytochrome by NADPH,

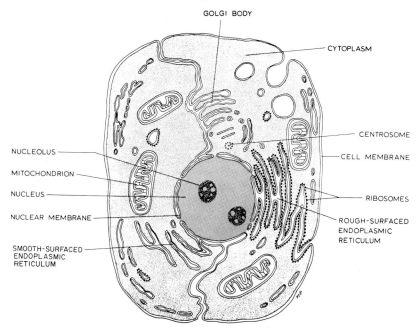

Figure 4–2   Schematic diagram of hepatocyte. The microsomal enzymes are located predominantly in liver cells, where they are associated primarily with the smooth-surfaced endoplasmic reticulum. (After concept of Robertson, J. D.: The membrane of the living cell. Copyright © 1962 by Scientific American, Inc. All rights reserved.)

suitably termed NADPH-cytochrome P-450 reductase. Cytochrome P-450 is also involved in the hydroxylation of lipid-soluble endogenous compounds, such as steroid hormones and fatty acids (ω-oxidation). The flavoprotein NADPH-cytochrome P-450 reductase most probably is closely related to the enzyme known as NADPH-cytochrome c reductase (Orrenius, 1971). The ability of the microsomal drug-metabolizing enzymes to mediate a wide variety of oxidation reactions may be ascribed to a common mechanism, hydroxylation (Brodie et al., 1958; Gillette, 1963, 1966). The mixed-function oxidase or monoxygenase (Hayaishi, 1962) mechanism requires that NADPH reduce a component, cytochrome P-450, in microsomes. The reduced cytochrome P-450 reacts with molecular oxygen to form an "active oxygen" intermediate. The "active oxygen" form of cytochrome P-450 decomposes into oxidized drug, oxidized P-450, and an equivalent of H_2O (Fig. 4–3). The overall reaction involves the oxidation of NADPH and the hydroxylation of the drug or steroid substrate. Substrates capable of undergoing hydroxylation bind to cytochrome P-450, and the reduction of the cytochrome

HEPATIC MICROSOMAL DRUG OXIDIZING SYSTEM

$$NADPH + A + H^+ \rightarrow AH_2 + NADP^+$$

$$AH_2 + O_2 \rightarrow \text{"active oxygen complex"}$$

$$\text{"active oxygen complex"} + drug \rightarrow oxidized\ drug + A + H_2O$$

This oxidative mechanism requires that equivalent amounts of NADPH, oxygen and drug substrate be utilized in the reaction.   A represents the oxidized form and AH_2 is the reduced form of cytochrome P-450.

Figure 4-3 Oxidation reaction catalyzed by the microsomal enzyme system.

Table 4-2 OXIDATIVE TRANSFORMATIONS CATALYZED BY THE LIVER MICROSOMAL ENZYME SYSTEM

Oxidative Reaction	Substrate	Metabolite
Aromatic hydroxylation	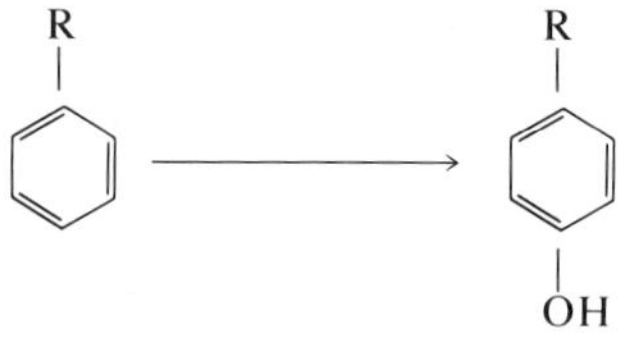	
	Amphetamine	*p*-Hydroxyamphetamine
	Phenobarbital	*p*-Hydroxyphenobarbital
	Acetanilide	Acetaminophen
	Phenylbutazone	Oxyphenbutazone
Side chain (aliphatic) oxidation	$R-CH_2-CH_3 \longrightarrow R-CH_2-CH_2OH$	
	$R-CH_2-CH_3 \longrightarrow R-CHOH-CH_3$	
	Pentobarbital	5-Ethyl-5(3'-hydroxy-1'-methylbutyl) Barbituric acid
Oxidative dealkylation: O-dealkylation	$R-O-CH_3 \rightarrow [R-O-CH_2OH] \rightarrow R-OH + HCHO$ unstable	
	Codeine	Morphine
	Phenacetin	Acetaminophen
	Trimethoprim	
	Griseofulvin	6-Demethylgriseofulvin

Table continued on opposite page

P-450–substrate complex so formed may well be the rate-limiting step in the overall hydroxylation process.

Species differences in activity of P-450 reductase have been shown to parallel differences in rates of drug oxidation (Davies et al., 1969). The oxidative reactions carried out by the liver microsomes are many and varied (Table 4–2) and include aromatic hydroxylation, oxidation of alkyl chains (aliphatic oxidation), O- and N-dealkylation, oxidative deamination, replacement of S by O, and sulfoxidation. The fate of most lipid-soluble foreign organic compounds introduced into the body is microsomal oxidation, which may be followed by glucuronide (and other) conjugation, along with renal excretion of some unchanged drug together with the metabolites. Amphetamine can be metabolized via two oxidation pathways, either by hydroxylation of the aromatic ring or by deamination of the side-chain (Fig. 4–4).

Table 4–2 OXIDATIVE TRANSFORMATIONS CATALYZED BY THE LIVER MICROSOMAL ENZYME SYSTEM (*Continued*)

Oxidative Reaction	Substrate	Metabolite
N-dealkylation	$R—R'N—CH_3 \rightarrow [R—R'N—CH_2OH] \rightarrow$ unstable	$R—R'NH + HCHO$
	where $R' = H$ or CH_3	
	Imipramine	Desmethylimipramine (desipramine)
	Diazepam	N-Desmethyldiazepam
Oxidative deamination	$R—CH(NH_2)—CH_3 \rightarrow [R—C(OH)(NH_2)—CH_3]$ $\downarrow$ $R—CO—CH_3 + NH_3$	
	Amphetamine	Phenylacetone
Replacement of S by O (*desulfuration*)	$\begin{array}{c} R \\ \diagdown \\ C{=}S \\ \diagup \\ R' \end{array} \longrightarrow \left[\begin{array}{c} R \\ \diagdown \\ C{=}S(OH) \\ \diagup \\ R' \end{array}\right]$ $\downarrow$ $\begin{array}{c} R \\ \diagdown \\ C{=}O + SH^- \\ \diagup \\ R \end{array}$	
	Parathion (P=S)	Paraoxon
	Thiopental (C=S)	Pentobarbital
Sulfoxidation	$R—S—R' \rightarrow [R—SOH—R^1]^+ \rightarrow R—SO—R^1 + H^+$	
	Chlorpromazine and other phenothiazines	Corresponding 5-oxides

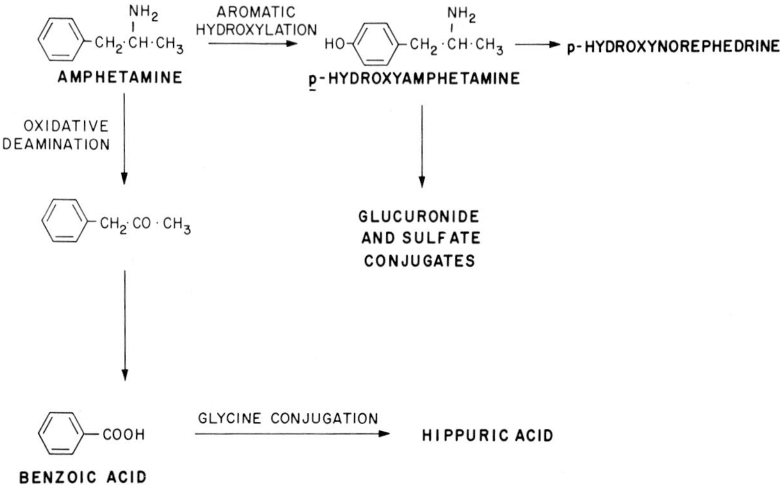

Figure 4-4 Metabolic pathways of amphetamine.

These two reactions have been demonstrated to take place and their relative extent appears to vary with the species of animal (Axelrod, 1954; Ellison et al., 1966; Dring et al., 1970; Baggot and Davis, 1973). In addition to unchanged drug in urine, the metabolites isolated were *p*-hydroxyamphetamine and benzoic acid, and their conjugates. Pronounced species differences in the metabolism of methylphenidate were found in humans, dogs, rats and mice (Faraj et al., 1974). The predominant route of metabolism of the drug in humans was via deesterification to ritalinic acid. In contrast to humans, microsomal oxidation represented a major route of metabolism of the drug in rats, mice and dogs *in vivo*. Phenacetin (acetophenetidin) and acetanilid are transformed in the body by the microsomal oxidative reactions O-dealkylation and aromatic hydroxylation, respectively, to acetaminophen (Brodie and Axelrod, 1948, 1949). This metabolite, which is more polar than either parent compound, is also a mild analgesic and antipyretic agent. Further metabolism of acetaminophen entails typical conjugation reactions (Fig. 4-5), yielding a sulfate ester and a glucuronide. Both conjugates, which are highly polar compounds, are pharmacologically inactive and are readily excreted in the urine.

The biotransformation of lidocaine, which is a local anesthetic agent and is also clinically effective in controlling ventricular arrhythmias, was studied in rats, guinea pigs, dogs and humans (Keenaghan and Boyes, 1972). Comparisons of the amount of lidocaine and its major metabolites excreted in 24-hour urine samples of the various

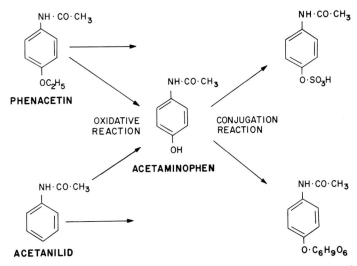

Figure 4–5 Biotransformation of phenacetin, acetanilid, and acetaminophen.

species indicate extensive biotransformation in all species and variations among species in the metabolic pattern (Table 4–3). The predominant route of metabolism in rats was via hydroxylation of the aromatic nucleus of lidocaine and the N-deethylated metabolite,

Table 4–3 SPECIES VARIATIONS IN THE METABOLISM
OF LIDOCAINE*

	Percentage of Dose Recovered in Urine†			
Compound	RAT	GUINEA PIG	DOG	MAN
Lidocaine	0.2	0.5	2.0	2.8
Monoethylglycinexylidide	0.7	14.9	2.3	3.7
Glycinexylidide	2.1	3.3	12.6	2.3
3-Hydroxylidocaine	31.2	0.5	6.7	1.1
3-Hydroxymonoethyl-glycinexylidide	36.9	2.0	3.1	0.3
2,6-Xylidine	1.5	16.2	1.6	1.0
4-Hydroxy-2,6-dimethyl-aniline	12.4	16.4	35.2	72.6
Total	85.0	53.8	63.5	83.8

*Data from Keenaghan and Boyes (1972): The tissue distribution, metabolism and excretion of lidocaine in rats, guinea pigs, dogs and man. *J. Pharmacol. exp. Ther.*, *180*:454–463. © 1972, The Williams and Wilkins Company, Baltimore.
†Doses and recovery fractions were quantitated as molar concentrations of the free bases.

monoethylglycinexylidide (Fig. 4–6). The other three species excreted much smaller quantities of these hydroxylated metabolites,
with dogs apparently having the most active hydroxylating ability of
the three. Both guinea pigs and dogs excrete approximately the same
total amount of N-dealkylated products (20 per cent) and products of
hydrolysis (about 35 per cent). The primary metabolic pathway in
humans was hydrolysis of the amide bond in lidocaine or one of its
dealkylated metabolites. Furthermore, the hydrolysis product was
excreted almost entirely as its hydroxylated metabolite.

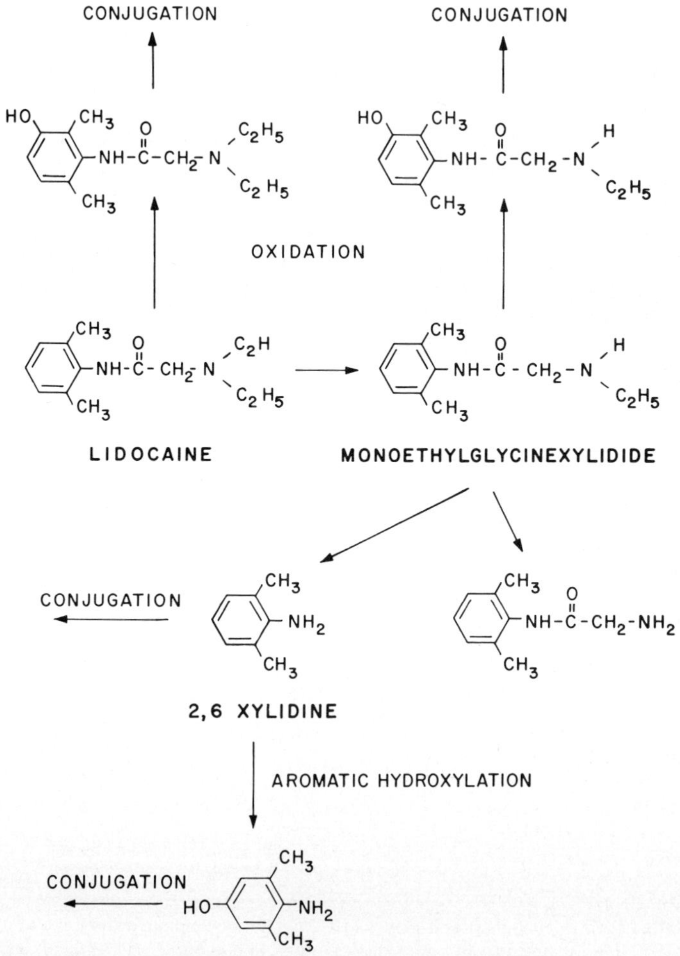

Figure 4–6 The metabolic fate of lidocaine. (From Keenaghan, J. B., and Boyes,
R. N. [1972]: The tissue distribution, metabolism and excretion of lidocaine in rats,
guinea pigs, dogs and man. *J. Pharmacol. exp. Ther.*, 180:454–463.)

In addition to catalyzing various oxidative reactions, the liver microsomes can reduce nitro- and azo-compounds to amines. The nitro-reductase enzyme system inactivates chloramphenicol. Interestingly, this metabolic reaction also takes place in the rumen, the significance of which is that the oral route of administration would be unsuitable for systemic therapy with chloramphenicol in ruminant animals.

The most common types of hydrolyses that occur in the body are of compounds with an ester ($-\overset{\overset{\textstyle O}{\|}}{C}-O-$) or an amide ($-\overset{\overset{\textstyle O}{\|}}{C}-NH-$) linkage. The hydrolytic reaction is an important metabolic pathway in the inactivation of some drugs and in the alteration in pharmacological activity of many others. Ester linkages occur in widely different types of drugs, such as local anesthetics (procaine, cocaine), narcotic analgesics (heroin, Pethidine, also called meperidine), insecticides (parathion, Malathion), the esters of choline (acetylcholine, neostigmine), atropine and acetylsalicylic acid (aspirin). The esterases are widely distributed, occurring not only in liver microsomes but also in the blood plasma and other tissues. Furthermore, these enzymes vary widely from tissue to tissue and within species and strains. Variations among the species of domestic animals in the dosage of succinylcholine required to produce neuromuscular block reflect species differences in activity of pseudocholinesterase. Relatively small doses of succinylcholine produce a desirable degree of blockade in dogs, sheep and cattle, whereas much higher doses are required in cats, pigs and horses (Tavernor, 1971). A low esterase activity in insects compared with that in mammals forms the basis of the selectively toxic action of organic phosphate insecticides (Loomis, 1968). Amides (e.g., procainamide, lidocaine) are hydrolyzed by amidases, which are found principally in the soluble fraction of the liver, but the reaction proceeds at a considerably slower rate than that of ester linkage hydrolysis.

It is appropriate at this point to state that foreign compounds can be metabolized (both phase I and phase II reactions) by other than microsomal enzyme systems. These metabolic reactions include deamination of amines, oxidation of alcohols and aldehydes, reduction of aldehydes and ketones, hydrolysis of esters and amides, and certain types of synthetic reactions (sulfate and glycine conjugation, acetylation).

Monoamine oxidase (MAO) is localized largely in the outer membrane of mitochondria and is found especially in liver, kidney, intestine and nerve tissue. This enzyme oxidatively deaminates catecholamines (dopamine, norepinephrine, epinephrine) and other biogenic amines such as 5-hydroxytryptamine (serotonin) and tyramine. The intraneuronal localization of MAO in mitochondria suggests that this would limit its action to amines that are present in a free (unbound) form in the axoplasm, that is, after the amines have been taken up by the axon but before they become bound in the granules. The enzyme converts catecholamines to their corresponding aldehydes. This aldehyde intermediate is rapidly metabolized to the corresponding acid, usually by oxidation catalyzed by aldehyde dehydrogenase. Extraneuronal metabolism of the catecholamines is mediated by catechol-O-methyltransferase (COMT). This enzyme is relatively nonspecific and catalyzes the transfer of methyl groups from S-adenosyl-methionine to the *m*-hydroxyl group of catecholamines and various other catechol compounds. Catechol-O-methyltransferase is found in the cytoplasm of most animal tissues, being particularly abundant in kidney and liver. A substantial amount of this enzyme is also found in the central nervous system and in various sympathetically innervated organs. Following release of norepinephrine and its action at adrenoceptive site of effector cells, the excess is efficiently removed from the extracellular region, largely by reuptake by the axonal terminal through active transport and, to some extent, by diffusion and subsequent enzymatic inactivation by mitochondrial MAO. Extraneuronal COMT also contributes to the termination of the effects of adrenergic impulses. Epinephrine and congeners (isoproterenol) administered parenterally are enzymatically inactivated by COMT and MAO; amines lacking the 3-OH group are unaffected by COMT, and their inactivation depends upon MAO (see Goodman and Gilman, 1975, Chapters 21 and 24).

An hypothesis involving catecholamine in the induction of affective disorders has arisen which states that, in general, behavioral depression may be related to a deficiency of catecholamine (usually norepinephrine) at functionally important central adrenergic receptors, whereas mania results from excess of catecholamine. The three general classes of drugs most commonly used to treat various depressive disorders are the MAO inhibitors (e.g., isocarboxazid, phenelzine and tranylcypromine), the tricyclic antidepressants (e.g., imipramine, desipramine, amitriptyline, and so forth), and the psychomotor stimulants, of which amphetamine is the prototype. All of these pharmacological agents appear to interact with catecholamines in a way that is consistent with the catecholamine hypothesis (Cooper et al., 1970).

Hepatic biotransformation accounts almost entirely for the fate of propranolol, a β-adrenergic receptor blocking drug. The initial pattern of biotransformation involves various oxidative reactions (Fig. 4–7). Both the parent drug and most metabolites are excreted in urine of humans and dogs as glucuronide and ethereal sulfate conjugates (Walle and Gaffney, 1972). Alcohol dehydrogenase and aldehyde

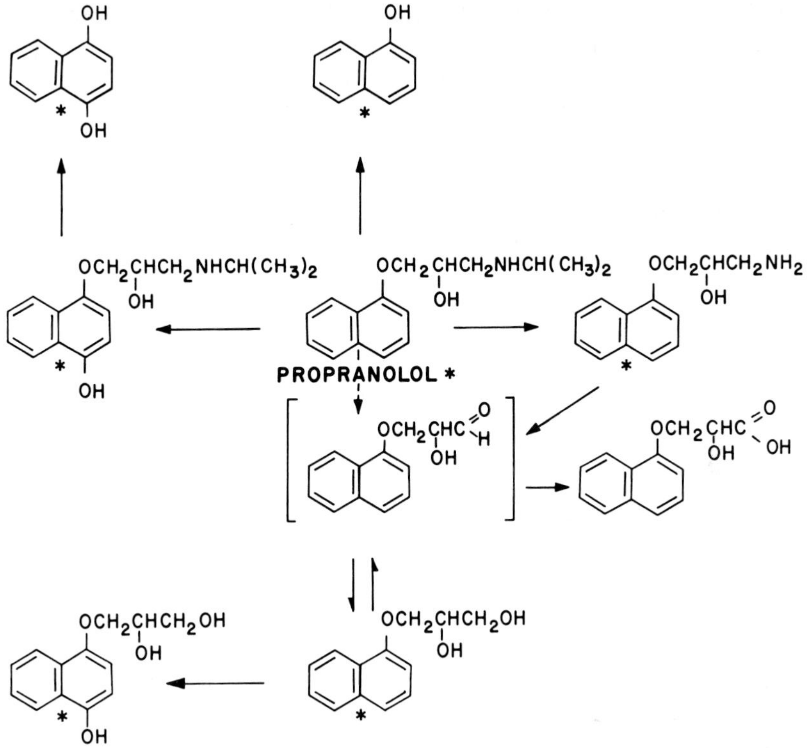

Figure 4–7 Schematic representation of propranolol metabolism in man and dog. Several of the metabolites appear to have pharmacological activity. Asterisk indicates the compounds which are excreted to a large extent as glucuronides and ethereal sulfates in the urine. (From Walle, T., and Gaffney, T. E. [1972]: *J. Pharmacol. exp. Ther.,* *182*:83–92.)

dehydrogenase are relatively nonspecific enzymes, found in the soluble fraction of liver, which catalyze several important oxidative transformations. The substrates include endogenous compounds (e.g., vitamin A and retinine, and catecholamines after oxidation by MAO), as well as some drugs (e.g., propranolol, ethanol, chloral hydrate). Alcohol dehydrogenase functions as a reductase when it catalyzes the conversion of chloral hydrate to the pharmacologically active (hypnotic) metabolite trichloroethanol (Friedman and Cooper, 1960; Mackay and Cooper, 1962). Intravenously administered chloral hydrate has an apparent half-life of 3 min in the dog, being rapidly and quantitatively converted to trichloroethanol (Garrett and Lambert, 1973). The major route of trichloroethanol removal is conjugation with glucuronic acid. The glucuronide, after release from the liver, is distributed only in the extracellular fluid and is rapidly eliminated by renal excretion (glomerular filtration and tubular excretion), with some biliary excretion.

Species variations usually are found in the biotransformation pattern of lipid-soluble compounds. Differences in the duration of action of these drugs in various species can frequently be attributed to differences in their rates of biotransformation. Knowledge of the metabolic pathways and rates of formation (which correspond to quantitative significance) of the various metabolites of a drug is necessary for the interpretation and application of data in development of drugs for clinical medicine. Variations in the nature and rate of formation of phase I metabolites may have considerable practical significance, as it is conceivable that a pharmacologically active metabolite could be quantitatively important in one species but not in others. Divergences between plasma levels and effects of a drug suggest the possibility of an active metabolite being formed from the administered drug. Phase I metabolic reactions appear to be ubiquitous in the animal kingdom, and predictable rankings (or patterns) among domestic or laboratory animals in the rates and even pathways of these reactions have not been discovered. One can expect to find marked interspecies differences in the metabolic fate of drugs, particularly if their biotransformation is mediated by the microsomal enzyme systems. Variations in the velocities of phase I metabolic reactions and in hepatic blood flow contribute significantly to species differences in drug biotransformation.

Phase II (Synthetic) Reactions

Synthetic reactions called conjugations may take place when the drug or phase I metabolite contains a chemical group such as hydroxyl (—OH), carboxyl (—COOH), amino (—NH$_2$) or sulfhydryl (—SH), which is suitable for combining with a natural compound provided by the body to form readily excreted water-soluble polar metabolites (Williams, 1971). The compounds provided by the body for conjugation (i.e., conjugating agents) are derived from materials involved in normal carbohydrate, protein and fat metabolism and include glucuronic acid, glycine, cysteine, methionine (for methylation), sulfate, acetic acid and thiosulfate (for sulfur). In anserine (duck, goose) and gallinaceous (hen, turkey) birds, ornithine replaces glycine in conjugation reactions. Almost without exception, conjugation reactions convert drugs and natural metabolites of the body into products that are pharmacologically and biologically inactive, respectively. This metabolic pathway not only inactivates drugs but also facilitates their removal from the body.

Table 4–4 ANIMAL SPECIES DEFECTIVE IN
CERTAIN CONJUGATION REACTIONS

Species	Conjugation	Major Target Groups	Extent of Synthetic Reaction
Cat	Glucuronide synthesis	—OH, —COOH, —NH$_2$, >NH, —SH	Low level
Dog	Acetylation	Ar—NH$_2$ R—NH—NH$_2$	Absent
Pig	Sulfate conjugation (ethereal sulfate formation)	Ar—OH Ar—NH$_2$	Low level
Domestic animals	Ornithine conjugation	Ar—COOH	Absent

Glycine conjugation takes place in animals and pigeons, whereas ornithine conjugation is the equivalent synthetic reaction in birds classified as gallinaceous (hen, turkey) and anserine (duck, goose) (Williams, 1967a).

A conjugation reaction requires, among other things, an "active" intermediate compound, usually a nucleotide, and a transferring enzyme. The mechanism of conjugation takes place in two stages. In the first stage, either the drug or the conjugating agent forms part of an "activated" nucleotide. In the second stage, the nucleotide reacts with the other component (drug or conjugating agent) of the conjugation system, under the influence of a transferring enzyme. Species variations in conjugation reactions can depend on the occurrence of the conjugating agent, the ability to form the necessary nucleotide or the amount of the transferring enzyme (Williams, 1971). In contrast to phase I metabolic reactions which occur at an unpredictable rate and to a variable degree among the species of domestic animals, certain phase II reactions are either deficient or absent in particular species (Table 4–4), so that a somewhat predictable metabolic pattern exists among the species.

Glucuronic Acid Conjugation

Glucuronic acid conjugation is an extremely important pathway of drug biotransformation. The reactive chemical groups for glucuronide synthesis are —OH, —COOH, —NH$_2$, and —SH (Dutton, 1966); compounds involved include alcohols, phenols, carboxylic acids (mainly aromatic), amines, amides and thiols. The conjugating agent is glucuronic acid ($C_6H_{10}O_6$), which is provided via glucose from the body's carbohydrate sources. Activation of glucuronic acid involves

Stage 1: Activation of glucuronic acid by formation of UDPGA

$$\text{Glucose-1-phosphate} + \text{Uridine triphosphate} \xrightarrow{\text{pyrophosphorylase}}$$
$$\text{Uridine diphosphate glucose} + \text{Pyrophosphate}$$

$$\text{Uridine diphosphate glucose} + 2\ NAD^+ + H_2O \xrightarrow[\text{dehydrogenase}]{\text{UDPG-}}$$
$$\text{Uridine diphosphate glucuronic acid (UDPGA)} + 2\ NADH + 2H^+$$

Stage 2: Transfer of conjugating agent from nucleotide UDPGA to drug

$$\text{Uridine diphosphate glucuronic acid} + RZH \xrightarrow[\text{transferase}]{\text{glucuronyl}} \begin{array}{l} RZ\text{-glucuronic} \\ \text{acid} + \text{Uridine} \\ \text{diphosphate} \end{array}$$

where $Z = O$, COO, NH or S

Figure 4–8   Mechanism of glucuronic acid conjugation.

the formation of uridine diphosphate glucuronic acid (UDPGA), which is mediated by enzymes in the soluble fraction of liver (Fig. 4–8). Synthesis of the glucuronide proceeds by way of transfer of glucuronic acid from the "activated" nucleotide (UDPGA) to an acceptor molecule; the transfer is catalyzed by the microsomal enzyme glucuronyl transferase (Isselbacher et al., 1962). The microsomal enzymes involved in glucuronide syntheses are unique in that this is the only conjugation reaction associated with microsomal enzymes, and a wide range of endogenous compounds (e.g., steroid hormones, thyroxine, bilirubin), as well as drugs and phase I metabolites, are substrates. Drugs that are conjugated with glucuronic acid include morphine, acetaminophen, salicylic acid, meprobamate, sulfadimethoxine, and chloramphenicol. The acquisition of a functional chemical group by a phase I reaction precedes glucuronide conjugation of most drugs.

Glucuronides are more water-soluble than the parent drugs because of the large hydrophilic carbohydrate moiety, and because of this the partition ratio between a lipid and an aqueous solvent is considerably reduced. Furthermore, the glucuronides are usually stronger acids than the parent drugs, and thus are more ionized at physiological pH values. Such compounds are less likely to diffuse across cellular membranes, so that their distribution will be restricted and their availability for excretion increased. Glucuronides of most drugs are excreted by the kidney by a combination of glomerular filtration and tubular excretion processes. In certain species, notably rats, dogs and chickens, the biliary route of excretion may predominate for glucuronide conjugates with molecular weights exceeding 400 (e.g., the glucuronides of bilirubin, diethylstilbestrol, morphine, chloramphenicol and sulfadimethoxine N[1]-glucuronide). In humans and monkeys, sulfadimethoxine N^1-glucuronide is the major metabolite of this drug and is excreted in the urine (Bridges et al., 1968). Compounds of molecular weight greater than 500 (e.g., indomethacin glucuronide, iopanoic acid [cholecystographic agent], Bromsulphalein) are excreted in bile of all mammalian species. Following passage of glucuronide conjugates into the gut, they may undergo hydrolysis mediated by intestinal β-glucuronidase with liberation of the aglycone and, if this parent compound is lipid-soluble, it will be reabsorbed (enterohepatic circulation). Although glucuronide conjugates of drugs are inactive, hydrolysis by β-glucuronidase restores activity (Smith and Williams, 1966).

Except in cats, glucuronide conjugation of drugs is a major metabolic pathway for the various species of domestic animals. In cats, the rate of synthesis of glucuronides is extremely slow compared with other species. It has been shown that cats can synthesize UDPGA, but apparently have deficient levels of glucuronyl transferases (Dutton, 1966). The limited capacity of this metabolic pathway in cats may increase the pharmacological response and the potential toxicity, and may lengthen the duration of action of lipid-soluble drugs. Since the fate of salicylate involves glucuronide formation, particular attention must be given to the dosage regimen for aspirin in cats. The acidity of the urine, which is characteristic of carnivorous species, promotes renal tubular reabsorption by nonionic diffusion of unchanged salicylate and contributes to the persistence of salicylate in cats. Various endogenous compounds, such as bilirubin, thyroxine and steroids, are conjugated as glucuronides in cats as well as in the other species. Goldfish and perch apparently do not form glucuronides (Brodie and Maickel, 1962), but conjugation of aminobenzoic acids with glucuronic acid has been reported to occur in some other species of fish (Adamson, 1967). The Gunn strain of Wistar rats is characteristic in its diminished ability to conjugate certain compounds with glucuronic acid. In insects, glucuronide formation is replaced by β-glucoside conjugation, the active conjugating agent is uridine diphosphate glucose (UDPG), and glucosyl transferases mediate transfer of the sugar moiety to a foreign compound (Parke, 1968).

Sulfate Conjugation

Phenolic and, to a much lesser extent, alcoholic compounds may be conjugated with sulfate to form sulfate esters, called ethereal sulfates. Synthesis of sulfamates is a minor reaction of aromatic amines (e.g., aniline). In the first stage of the conjugation reaction sulfate is activated by a series of reactions involving ATP and resulting in formation of 3'-phosphoadenosine-5'-phosphosulfate (PAPS). Relatively specific sulfokinases mediate the second stage of the conjugation process, which is the reaction between PAPS and the hydroxyl group of phenols. Both stages of sulfate conjugation are catalyzed by enzymes which are found in the soluble fraction of liver cells (Robbins and Lipmann, 1957; Nose and Lipmann, 1958). Phenolic compounds which form ethereal sulfates include phenol, acetaminophen, morphine, isoproterenol and 3-hydroxycoumarin. Various endogenous substances, such as chondroitin sulfate, numerous steroids and bile acids are known to form sulfate esters. The ethereal sulfates appear to be more water-soluble than their parent compounds and are readily excreted in the urine. Formation of the sulfate esters of phenolic compounds is widespread among species (Smith, 1968). The pig, however, appears to synthesize ethereal sulfates less readily than other species (Stekol, 1936). The sulfate pool in the body is quite limited and can be easily exhausted; conjugation with glucuronic acid usually predominates over sulfate formation.

Acetylation

Acetylation of OH (e.g., choline) and SH (e.g., CoA—SH) has been shown to occur *in vivo* for natural compounds, but for drugs the acetylation of NH_2 is the only important reaction of this type. At least five types of amino groups that can be acetylated *in vivo* are distinguishable, and this may indicate the existence of several N-acetylases (Williams, 1967a). The active conjugating agent is acetyl-CoA, which reacts with free amino groups on the drug to form an amide bond, catalyzed by transacetylases. Acetylation is the primary route of biotransformation for the sulfonamide compounds. In a number of species, including humans but not dogs, sulfanilamide gives rise to three acetyl derivatives, namely N^1-monoacetyl-, N^4-monoacetyl-, and N^1,N^4-diacetylsulfanilamide (Fig. 4–9). The dog and fox were the only species in which acetylation of the aromatic amino group (Ar—NH_2) of sulfanilamide does not take place, whereas the sulfamoyl group (Ar—SO_2NH_2) was acetylated in all of the several species studied (Williams, 1967a). The selectivity of the acetylation reaction for various types of amino groups suggests an enzyme specificity of the transacetylases. The acetylation reaction takes place in the reticuloendothelial, rather than parenchymal, cells of the liver, spleen, lungs and intestinal mucosa (Govier, 1965). Phenols, alcohols or thiol drugs do not form acetyl derivatives, although certain natural compounds with such functional groups, such as choline and coenzyme A, react in this manner. Acetylation of most sulfonamide compounds exemplifies the point that a decrease in lipid-solubility does not neces-

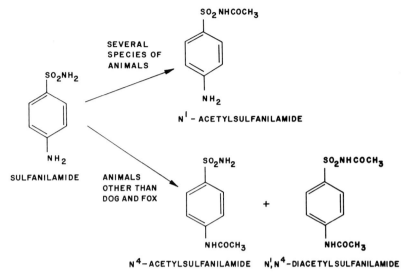

Figure 4–9   Acetylation reactions of sulfanilamide in several species of animals. The dog and fox are unable to form the N^4-acetyl derivative.

sarily mean an increase in water-solubility. The solubility of sulfa-thiazole, for example, is 98 mg per 100 ml water at 37° C, whereas its acetylated derivative is soluble to the extent of only 7 mg per 100 ml. As a result of the decrease in aqueous solubility, the acetylated de-rivatives have a greater tendency to precipitate in the renal tubules (crystalluria). Acetylation of sulfapyrimidines (e.g., sulfamethazine) in-creases their solubilities in water. The solubility of a sulfonamide and its acetyl derivative in urine decreases considerably with decrease in urinary pH. Solubility of sulfisoxazole in urine decreases from 14,500 to 150 mg per 100 ml and that of acetylsulfisoxazole decreases from 10,000 to 55 mg per 100 ml at urinary pH of 7.5 and 5.5 respectively. Urinary alkalinization increases both the solubility of sulfonamides and the proportion of the dose that is excreted unchanged in urine.

Procainamide is eliminated by a combination of renal excretion (glomerular filtration and tubular secretion) and biotransformation processes (Galeazzi et al., 1976). Although plasma esterases play a key role in the biotransformation of procaine, this is not the case for procainamide (Dreyfuss et al., 1971). In the dog, over 50 per cent of the dose is excreted unchanged in the urine as procainamide. The major metabolite was characterized as having an alteration of the aromatic amino group, but this was not the N-acetyl derivative. For-mation of N-acetyl procainamide is the principal metabolic pathway in the fate of procainamide in humans and Rhesus monkeys (Giardina et al., 1976; Dreyfuss et al., 1971). Reports in the literature indicate that N-acetyl procainamide has antiarrhythmic effects in animals (Drayer et al., 1974) and probably also in humans (Elson et al., 1975).

Methylation

A methyl group ($—CH_3$) derived from the amino acid methionine can be transferred from the active conjugating agent S-adenosylmethionine to a phenolic hydroxyl group, to a sulfydryl group or to various amino groups. The nitrogen atom in aromatic nitrogen heterocyclic compounds can also be methylated *in vivo*, to give rise to a quaternary nitrogen cation. Transfer of the methyl group from the intermediate nucleotide, S-adenosylmethionine, to the acceptor compound is catalyzed by various methyl transferases. Species variations in methylation could arise from differences in the occurrence and amounts of these transferases. The methylation of free or substituted amino groups has been observed mainly with endogenous amines containing aliphatic groups, such as norepinephrine and dimethylaminoethanol. In the adrenal medulla, norepinephrine is N-methylated by the enzyme phenylethanolamine-N-methyltransferase (PNMT) to form epinephrine. PNMT, which is abundant in the soluble fraction of the adrenal medulla, can methylate phenylethanolamines but not phenylethylamines.

N-Methylation (e.g., norepinephrine to epinephrine) can be written as:

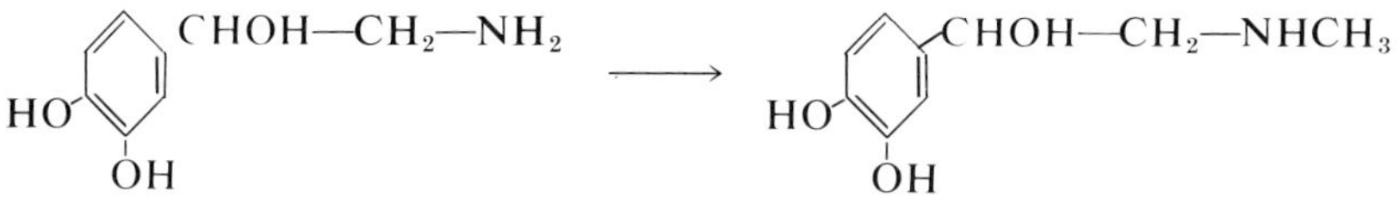

O-Methylation is a reaction of catechols (the catechol nucleus consists of a benzene ring with two adjacent hydroxyl substituents), but only one hydroxyl is methylated, usually the one which is *meta* to a substituent (Williams, 1967*b*). Catechol-O-methyl transferase (COMT), which is widely distributed in tissues, can catalyze the transfer of a methyl group to a phenolic hydroxyl group of epinephrine, norepinephrine and other catechol derivatives. This enzyme is involved in the inactivation of the adrenergic neurotransmitter norepinephrine, as well as other catecholamines, whether of endogenous or exogenous origin.

O-Methylation (e.g., epinephrine to metanephrine) can be exemplified by:

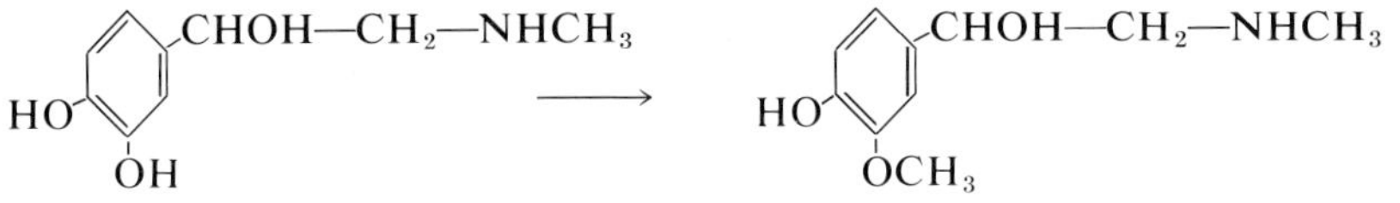

CHOH—CH$_2$—NHCH$_3$

HO

OH

$\longrightarrow$

CHOH—CH$_2$—NHCH$_3$

HO

OCH$_3$

Other important endogenous compounds that are methylated include histamine and the hormones estradiol and thyroxine. Methylation usually represents a relatively minor metabolic pathway for drugs (e.g., nicotinamide, quinidine).

In addition to methylation, demethylation can also take place. Methyl groups can be removed oxidatively by liver microsomes when they are attached through oxygen, nitrogen or sulfur. Examples of the O-demethylation reaction include conversion of codeine (3-methyl-morphine) to morphine, and of griseofulvin to 6-demethylgriseofulvin. The rapid biotransformation of trimethoprim in domestic animals compared with humans may be attributed in part to more efficient O-demethylation. The conversion of imipramine to desmethylimipramine (desipramine) is an N-demethylation reaction. Whereas oxidative demethylation is a phase I reaction, methylation is a phase II synthetic reaction.

Cyanide Detoxication

In the conjugation of cyanide to form thiocyanate, the donor of sulfur is thiosulfate, and the reaction is catalyzed by the mitochondrial enzyme sulfur transferase (formerly called "rhodanese"):

$$CN^- + S_2O_3^= \longrightarrow SCN^- + SO_3^=$$
cyanide   thiosulfate   thiocyanate   sulfite

Thiosulfate sulfur transferase is found in liver, kidney and other tissues, but very little is present in blood. The cyanide ion is normally converted *in vivo* to the innocuous thiocyanate (involving a 200-fold reduction in toxicity) by the reaction shown above. However, the rate of this reaction is ordinarily slow because the requisite sulfur donors (such as thiosulfate) are present in the body in limited amounts.

Cyanide combines with the ferric iron atom in heme proteins in the tissues, destroying their capacity to undergo oxidation and reduction in the normal electron transport process. Since in cyanide poisoning death can occur extremely rapidly, primarily by inactivation of cytochrome oxidase in tissues, the success of antidotal therapy depends largely upon the length of time between onset of intoxication and initiation of treatment. The first aim of treatment is to bind as much cyanide as possible in an inert form. This is accomplished by converting a proportion of the blood hemoglobin to methemoglobin, thus making a large amount of ferric heme available for interaction with cyanide. Methemoglobin is formed by injecting sodium nitrite intravenously. Methemoglobinemia itself does not present serious problems until more than half the available hemoglobin is converted to the non-oxygen-carrying form; however, conversion of about 50 per cent of hemoglobin yields enough methemoglobin to combine with more than a fatal dose of cyanide. The metabolic conversion of cyanide to thiocyanate can be accelerated by administering sodium thiosulfate. Thus, antidotal therapy of cyanide intoxication consists of administering sodium nitrite intravenously followed immediately by sodium thiosulfate. Administration of oxygen is also beneficial.

Metabolic Transformations Mediated by Gastrointestinal Microorganisms

The intestinal microorganisms can metabolize drugs and other foreign compounds (Scheline, 1968). Hydrolytic and reductive reactions are the usual types of metabolic transformations that are mediated by the gut microflora (Williams, 1972). These reactions include the hydrolysis of glucuronides, dehydroxylation of certain catechols, dealkylation, dehalogenation, deamination and reductions of various kinds. Bacterial metabolism may occur after oral administration of a compound or as a consequence of passive diffusion of lipid-soluble compounds from the systemic circulation into gastrointestinal fluids. Certain drugs or their metabolites, in particular glucuronide conjugates, of moderately high molecular weight (over 400) may be excreted via the bile into the intestine. Hydrolysis of a drug conjugate by the gut flora will liberate the active drug, which may be reabsorbed or be inactivated by reduction. The enterohepatic circulation of a compound may contribute to its persistence in the body. The marked differences among domestic animals in digestive physiology, as well as the nature and location of microorganisms within the gastrointestinal tract, must be considered when the oral route of drug administration is employed, since these can contribute to species variations in the fate of drugs.

Rate of Drug Metabolism

Studies of drug metabolism in living animals have made it possible to elucidate the metabolic pathways and the factors which control the levels of drugs and their metabolites at receptor sites. Without corollary *in vitro* studies, however, the interpretation of many *in vivo* studies would be virtually impossible (Gillette, 1971a).

Metabolism of drugs is described by Michaelis-Menten enzyme kinetics. The sequence of an enzyme-catalyzed reaction was envisaged as follows:

$$
\begin{array}{c}
k_1 \\
\text{Enzyme} + \text{Substrate} \rightleftarrows \text{Enzyme-Substrate Complex} \\
k_2 \qquad\qquad\qquad \downarrow k_3 \\
\text{Enzyme} + \text{Products}
\end{array}
$$

According to the Michaelis-Menten equation, the velocity of an enzyme reaction (v) or rate of metabolism is defined by:

$$ v = \frac{V_{max} \cdot [S]}{K_m + [S]} \qquad\qquad \textbf{Equation 4 • 1} $$

where [S] is the substrate concentration or concentration of a drug in blood plasma. V_{max} is the maximum velocity, and K_m is the Michaelis constant for the given substrate-enzyme system. By definition, K_m is that concentration of substrate which gives one-half the maximal rate of the reaction under the conditions of the assay. Although the drug concentration at the site of biotransformation is the substrate concentration of the enzyme-catalyzed reaction, *in vivo* studies of drug metabolism rates involve the assumption that drug concentrations in blood plasma and at site of biotransformation are proportional. This assumption is valid when biotransformation takes place in a highly perfused organ, such as liver.

The Michaelis-Menten equation may be rearranged to form a number of linear equations, which may be used to evaluate the apparent K_m and the apparent V_{max}. The most popular transformation is the Lineweaver-Burk (1934) procedure, on which is based the double-reciprocal plot. The relevant equation is:

$$ \frac{1}{v} = \frac{K_m}{V_{max}} \cdot \frac{1}{[S]} + \frac{1}{V_{max}} \qquad\qquad \textbf{Equation 4 • 2} $$

A graph of $1/v$ against $1/[S]$ yields a straight line, the slope of the line is K_m/V_{max} and the intercept on the Y axis is $1/V_{max}$ (Fig. 4–10). Extrapolation of the line to the X axis gives an intercept of $-1/K_m$. Although this type of plot has been widely used, it is probably the most inaccurate of the plotting techniques, because data obtained at low substrate concentrations are given more weight than data obtained at high substrate concentrations, even though data obtained at low substrate concentrations are usually less accurate. Moreover, the Lineweaver-Burk plot frequently fails to detect curvature of the line. Because of the statistical inaccuracies of the double-reciprocal plot, the $[S]/v$ versus $[S]$ plot, also suggested by Lineweaver and Burk (1934), has gained increasing popularity. This plot is described by the equation:

$$\frac{[S]}{v} = \frac{[S]}{V_{max}} + \frac{K_m}{V_{max}}$$

Equation 4 • 3

A graph of $[S]/v$ against $[S]$ gives a straight line, the slope is $1/V_{max}$ and the intercept on the Y axis is K_m/V_{max}. When the line is extrapolated to the X axis the intercept is $-K_m$ (Fig. 4–10). Although this type of plot (sometimes called the Woolf plot) weights the data ob-

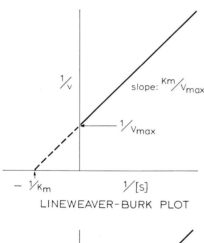

LINEWEAVER-BURK PLOT

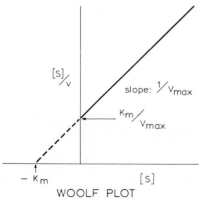

WOOLF PLOT

Figure 4–10 Some graphic techniques to evaluate K_m and V_{max} for a given enzyme-substrate system.

tained at low and high substrate concentrations about equally, it still frequently fails to detect curvature of the line.

The Hofstee plot (1956) is based on equation:

$$v = V_{max} - K_m \cdot \left\{ \frac{v}{[S]} \right\} \qquad \text{Equation 4 • 4}$$

On plotting v versus $v/[S]$ the intercept on the Y axis is V_{max}, the slope is $-K_m$ and the intercept on the X axis is V_{max}/K_m (Fig. 4–11). This plot weights the data obtained at low and high substrate concentrations about equally. Its principal advantage, however, is that it will detect curvature of the line. The Scatchard plot (1949), which is widely used to measure binding of substances to plasma albumin, is based on an analogous equation.

Within the dose range of many therapeutic agents, only a small fraction of the total available metabolic sites are occupied. In other words, the substrate concentration is negligible in comparison with K_m, and [S] can be eliminated from the denominator of the Michaelis-Menten equation, which reduces to:

$$\text{Rate of metabolism} = \frac{d[S]}{dt} = \frac{V_{max}}{K_m} \cdot [S] \qquad \text{Equation 4 • 5}$$

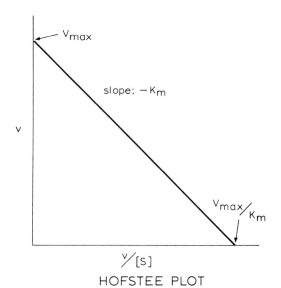

HOFSTEE PLOT

Figure 4–11   The Hofstee plot has certain advantages over Lineweaver-Burk and Woolf plots, but K_m is not as easily determined by this plot.

which is the equation of a first-order process, since V_{max}/K_m is a constant, with units of volume per unit time. Under these circumstances, metabolism is a first-order process; that is, the rate of metabolism is directly proportional to the concentration of the drug. This situation prevails for many drugs when therapeutic doses are administered.

Some drugs can saturate the metabolizing enzyme system, even within the therapeutic range of plasma levels, so that their metabolic inactivation is constant in rate and practically independent of the concentration in plasma. Under these conditions, it is K_m which is effectively negligible and can be eliminated from the denominator of the Michaelis-Menten equation. Thus, the rate of metabolism becomes maximal and is constant. An important consequence of zero-order metabolism is that the pharmacological effect is disproportionately prolonged with increasing dose. As the drug concentration declines, a level is reached at which the kinetics of metabolism change from a zero-order to a first-order process. Initially, therefore, biotransformation (and overall elimination) of a drug may be zero-order or first-order, depending upon the drug concentration and on the affinity of the drug for its metabolizing enzymes. Eventually, as drug levels fall, biotransformation will become first-order.

Table 4–5   PROBABLE BIOTRANSFORMATION PATHWAYS
OF DRUGS WITH FUNCTIONAL GROUPS

Aromatic rings:	Hydroxylation
Hydroxyl (—OH):	
Aliphatic:	Chain oxidation; glucuronic acid conjugation; (sulfate conjugation)
Aromatic:	Glucuronic acid conjugation; sulfate conjugation; methylation
Carboxyl (—COOH):	
Aliphatic:	Glucuronic acid conjugation
Aromatic:	Glycine conjugation; glucuronic acid conjugation
Amino (—NH₂):	
Aliphatic:	Deamination
Aromatic:	Acetylation; glucuronic acid conjugation; methylation; (sulfate conjugation)
Sulfhydryl (—SH):	Glucuronic acid conjugation; methylation; oxidation

Drugs with an ester linkage $\left(\begin{array}{c} O \\ \parallel \\ -C-O- \end{array}\right)$ (e.g., aspirin, procaine, atropine) or an amide linkage $\left(\begin{array}{c} O\ \ H \\ \parallel\ \ | \\ -C-N- \end{array}\right)$ (e.g., lidocaine, procainamide, phthalylsulfathiazole) may undergo hydrolysis.

The nature of the functional groups determines the metabolic fate of a foreign organic compound (Table 4–5). Species variations in drug biotransformation are largely the result of differences in the rates of similar metabolic reactions. These differences in rates of metabolism are reflected quantitatively by the relative amounts of the various metabolites which are excreted in cumulative (usually 24 hour) urine samples. However, there can be, in addition, qualitative differences in the actual pathways of biotransformation. Whereas tissue enzymes are mainly responsible for species variations in drug biotransformation, the gastrointestinal flora can influence the overall metabolic pattern.

Drug-Induced Changes in Drug Metabolism

The duration of action of many drugs is determined by their rate of biotransformation by hepatic and possibly other microsomal enzymes. Enzymatic activity converts a nonpolar drug to a polar metabolite, usually renders drugs pharmacologically inert and provides a compound which is efficiently excreted. The activities of the hepatic microsomal drug-metabolizing enzymes are markedly enhanced when animals are treated with a variety of drugs, certain hormones, insecticides and carcinogens (Conney, 1967). This increase in enzymatic activity appears to represent an increased concentration of enzyme protein and is referred to as "enzyme induction." Enhanced activity, or induction, of liver microsomal enzymes leads to an accelerated biotransformation and alteration (usually a decrease) in the intensity and duration of the pharmacological effects of the inducing agent and of other concurrently administered drugs that are substrates for microsomal biotransformation reactions. Enzyme induction is also of physiological significance, since endogenous compounds, such as cortisol, bilirubin and the sex steroids, are substrates for inducible drug-metabolizing enzymes (Conney et al., 1965). Any drug that is lipid-soluble at physiological pH should be considered as being capable of inducing microsomal enzymes. Some therapeutic agents that are known to be enzyme-inducers are listed in Table 4–6. Chronic administration of either phenobarbital or phenylbutazone to dogs increases the rate of their metabolism. Enzyme induction usually develops over a period of several days or weeks, and persists for a similar period following withdrawal of the inducing agent. The effects of chlorinated hydrocarbon insecticides, such as DDT, are more persistent, since these chemical agents are stored in body fat and only slowly become available for interaction with drug-metabolizing enzymes. Chronic administration of low doses of phenobarbital to dairy cows given DDT for 2 months resulted in a significant decrease in the content of DDT-

Table 4–6   DRUGS THAT STIMULATE
MICROSOMAL ENZYME ACTIVITY

Inducing Agent	Class of Drug	Compounds Whose Rate of Biotransformation is Increased
Phenobarbital	Sedative	Barbiturates Phenytoin Phenylbutazone Bishydroxycoumarin Warfarin Cortisol Testosterone Progesterone Bilirubin
Phenylbutazone	Anti-inflammatory agent	Phenylbutazone Corticosteroids Sex steroids
Phenytoin	Anticonvulsant	Corticosteroids Sex steroids
Griseofulvin	Antifungal agent	Warfarin
Meprobamate	Sedative	Meprobamate Warfarin
Chlorinated hydrocarbons (DDT, Aldrin, Dieldrin)	Insecticide	Corticosteroids Sex steroids Thyroxine
Chloral hydrate	Hypnotic (pro-drug)	Bishydroxycoumarin Warfarin

related substances in the milk (Alary et al., 1971). Stimulation of the metabolism of coumarin anticoagulants (e.g., warfarin) by barbiturates or other hypnotics is one of the most important induction interactions in human beings. This effect requires that the dosage of coumarins be increased to maintain an adequate anticoagulant response; serious toxicity can result when the inducing agent is withdrawn and administration of the anticoagulant is continued without an appropriate decrease in dose.

Drug interactions are the sequelae attending the simultaneous use of two or more drugs. The consequences of enzyme induction for the animal depend upon the relative activity of a drug and its metabolites. Whenever microsomal enzymes convert a drug to inactive metabolites, enzyme induction will have the effect of decreasing activity of the therapeutic agent. Some drugs are converted to compounds of greater pharmacological activity, and certain drugs (e.g., Malathion) require biotransformation for activity. In such cases the induction of microsomal enzymes by the concomitant use of another drug may lead to increased pharmacological effects or even toxicity caused by the active metabolites.

Another type of drug interaction involves inhibition of the metabolism of one drug by another causing delayed elimination. Cumulation will occur, which is manifested by an exaggerated pharmacological response, and the increase in potential toxicity depends on the therapeutic index and efficiency of alternate routes for elimination of the drug. Delayed biotransformation may involve liver microsomal enzymes, and mechanisms include substrate competition, interference with drug transport, depletion of hepatic glycogen, and functional impairment of enzyme activity due to hepatotoxicity. Drugs that inhibit microsomal enzyme activity in animals include organophosphorus insecticides, pesticide synergists of the methylenedioxyphenyl type (e.g., piperonyl butoxide), quinidine, carbon tetrachloride and chloramphenicol. Compounds that inhibit drug-metabolizing enzymes in liver microsomes impair the metabolism of endogenous steroids.

Drug interactions based on inhibition of metabolism could be due to inactivation of an enzyme system responsible for drug biotransformation or be caused by substrate competition for the same drug-metabolizing enzyme. When the metabolic reaction obeys first-order kinetics, it is unlikely that substrate competition for the metabolizing enzymes will significantly delay inactivation. An important corollary, however, is that significant mutual inhibition of drug metabolism is to be expected for drugs that normally exhibit zero-order inactivation kinetics. Minor reactions may be responsible for adverse reactions to drugs, and these pathways may be stimulated or inhibited by the simultaneous administration of another drug or exposure to an environmental chemical (Conney and Burns, 1972). Alterations in plasma drug half-lives during thyroid dysfunction appear to result mainly from accelerated hepatic microsomal drug metabolism in hyperthyroidism and retarded drug biotransformation during hypothyroidism (Vesell et al., 1975b).

Some drugs inhibit nonmicrosomal enzymes that are responsible for inactivation of other drugs and some endogenous substances (e.g., catecholamines). Plasma pseudocholinesterase is irreversibly inactivated by organophosphorus insecticides. The monoamine oxidase inhibitors (e.g., pargyline and tranylcypromine) interact with many drugs. During MAO inhibition, the administration of catecholamine-releasing drugs (e.g., sympathomimetic agents) and consumption of natural products that are rich in tyramine may produce fatal hypertensive reactions (Brownlee and Williams, 1963; Horwitz et al., 1964;

Sjoqvist, 1965). The effects of tyramine, a primary phenolic amine found frequently in naturally fermented dairy and grape products, are normally transient because of rapid oxidation catalyzed by MAO. The MAO inhibitors have little or no potentiating action upon the cardiovascular effects of the natural catecholamines, presumably because tissue uptake and O-methylation rather than oxidative de-amination are primarily responsible for terminating their peripheral actions. Enzyme systems other than MAO may be nonspecifically inhibited during therapy with these drugs, accounting at least in part for the enhanced effects of sedatives, narcotics, tricyclic (imipramine) antidepressants, phenothiazines and hypoglycemic agents (Sjoqvist, 1965). Disulfiram (tetraethylthiuram disulfide) inhibits aldehyde dehydrogenase, the enzyme that normally oxidizes acetaldehyde to acetic acid in the detoxication pathway for ethanol. This compound also acts as a nonspecific inhibitor of microsomal drug-metabolizing enzymes (Stripp et al., 1969, Vesell et al., 1971).

Liver Disease and Drug Therapy

Liver disease comprises an assortment of inflammatory or degenerative lesions, and any of the several synthetic and metabolic functions, biliary excretory ability and hepatic blood flow can be abnormal. Whereas any of these factors can have effects on drug disposition, the activity of the hepatic microsomal drug-metabolizing enzymes will influence biotransformation of most lipid-soluble drugs. The response evoked by a drug given according to the usual dosage regimen may be enhanced in an animal with liver disease. The increased pharmacological activity may be due to a reduced rate of biotransformation, a decrease in the fraction bound to plasma proteins (which can be attributed to hypoalbuminemia) or a reduced hepatic blood flow.

The hepatic clearance of highly extracted drugs (e.g., lidocaine) is essentially perfusion-limited (Wilkinson, 1975). Congestive heart failure results in a decreased hepatic clearance of a number of compounds, and this is probably related to the perfusion changes that occur in the splanchnic circulation. It is difficult to separate the relative contributions of blood flow and extraction in an observed impairment of hepatic clearance when considering the effect of liver disease on the metabolism of drugs that normally have a high extraction ratio, for example lidocaine (Thomson et al., 1973) and meperidine (Klotz et al., 1974). A reduction in blood volume as a result of shock of varying etiology has a profound effect on hemodynamics, and drastic alterations in hepatic clearance can occur. Again, problems arise in attributing the latter to perfusion changes, which alter drug delivery and extraction, or to reduced oxygen supply to the liver and the mixed-function oxidase system(s). One drug may alter the rate of elimination of another by changing the rate of delivery to its site of elimination. The half-life of lidocaine in the dog was increased 50 per cent when dl-propranolol was administered. No discernible change occurred in the extraction ratio (which is the fraction of drug entering the liver that is cleared by elimination processes), but hepatic clearance, cardiac output and liver blood flow were significantly reduced (Branch et al., 1973). Since the pharmacologically inactive d-isomer caused no change in any of the above parameters, the prolongation of the half-life was ascribed to the alterations in hemodynamics. The differences in total body clearance of propranolol in humans (15 ml/kg/min) and dogs (34 ml/kg/min) have been explained on the basis of interspecies variation in hepatic perfusion rather than in biotransformation rate of this drug (Evans et al., 1973). The measured liver blood flow was 22 and 43 ml/kg/min in humans and dogs, respectively. Consideration should therefore be given to the organ perfusion characteristics in comparative drug metabolism studies.

There are two distinct approaches to studying the biotransformation of drugs by the diseased liver. One is by measuring the activity of drug-metabolizing enzymes in liver biopsies, and the other is by determining the disposition kinetics of drugs in patients with liver disease. There is no single *in vivo* test that can measure the activities of hepatic microsomal drug-metabolizing enzyme systems. In the dog, the half-life of antipyrine reflects the activity of a few, but not all, of these enzyme systems (Vesell et al., 1973).

Liver microsomal enzyme systems are routinely employed to study the extent and rate of drug metabolism and to determine what effect factors such as enzyme stimulators, enzyme inhibitors and various disease states may have on this metabolic activity (Gillette, 1971b; Remmer, 1972; Rosso et al., 1971; Rumack et al., 1973). In liver biopsies from patients with severe hepatitis and cirrhosis, a reduction in the content of cytochrome P-450 was demonstrated, together with a lowering of the demethylating activity of the drug-metabolizing enzymes (Schoene et al., 1972). NADPH cytochrome *c* reductase was normal in all of these patients. Measurement of enzyme activity in liver biopsy samples is useful but is probably of limited value in predicting the rates of biotransformation reactions *in vivo*, as the *in vitro* systems do not take into account hepatic blood flow or the total hepatic capacity for drug metabolism and disregard the supply of NADPH in the intact hepatocyte.

There is conflicting evidence in the literature regarding the effect of liver disease on the overall rate of elimination of some drugs that undergo extensive hepatic metabolism. The inconsistency of results is due mainly to lack of reliable methods for quantitative estimation of reduced liver function. The galactose elimination capacity may be the best method available for estimating the functioning liver mass (Tygstrup, 1964). A significant correlation was obtained between the apparent elimination rate constant of phenylbutazone (the plasma half-life) and the galactose elimination capacity ($r=0.868$, $p<0.05$) in cirrhotic patients (Hvidberg et al., 1974). The half-life values of chloramphenicol (Kunin et al., 1959) and meprobamate (Held and Oldershausen, 1969) are prolonged in patients with impaired hepatic function. It has been suggested that a correlation may exist in human liver disease between albumin synthesis and cytochrome P-450–dependent drug oxidation (Levi et al., 1968; Mawer et al., 1972).

Although dependent on various factors, a lower serum albumin seems to reflect reasonably well the severity and chronicity of hepatic parenchymal damage (Muting and Reikowski, 1965). Whether it is truly reflective of reduced microsomal enzyme activity is questionable. The half-life of phenobarbital is moderately prolonged in patients with cirrhosis (Alvin et al., 1975). Because of the important contribution of urinary excretion of unchanged phenobarbital to overall elimination of the drug from the body, the difference in mean half-life between the control and cirrhotic groups was only modest. The decreased rate of elimination in cirrhotics is most likely the result of impaired delivery of phenobarbital into the liver or reduced hydroxylation of the drug within the liver, or both. Decreased urinary excretion of the glucuronide conjugate is probably reflective of diminished production of the *p*-hydroxy derivative. *In vitro* studies of glucuronyl transferase activity for bilirubin in cirrhosis failed to show impaired activity of this enzyme (Black and Billing, 1969).

Hepatic drug-metabolizing enzyme activity in man is commonly assessed by measurement of the plasma antipyrine (phenazone) half-life (Prescott et al., 1973). Antipyrine is particularly well suited for this purpose since it is well absorbed after oral administration, rapidly and evenly distributed in total body water (Soberman et al., 1949), does not bind to tissue proteins, and is excreted in urine entirely as conjugated metabolite (Brodie and Axelrod, 1950). Consequently, elimination of antipyrine from the plasma is dependent primarily on its rate of metabolism by liver microsomal enzymes. In therapeutic doses antipyrine is safe and produces no subjective pharmacological effects. Compounds that inhibit the drug-metabolizing system in the liver prolong markedly the plasma half-life of antipyrine (Vesell et al., 1970, 1971, 1972), and compounds that enhance the metabolism of drugs by liver significantly shorten the plasma half-life of antipyrine (Cucinell et al., 1965; Conney et al., 1967; Welch et al., 1967; Kolmodin et al., 1969). Moreover, the rate of excretion of the metabolite, 4-hydroxyantipyrine, in urine correlates well with the rate of disappearance of antipyrine from plasma (Huffman et al., 1974). The correlation is actually between the half-life of antipyrine as determined from plasma and urinary data (Vesell et al., 1975a). The distribution ratio of antipyrine between saliva and plasma is essentially 1 in rats and humans (no binding to plasma proteins) following administration of an oral or parenteral dose of the drug, so that the elimination rate of antipyrine may be determined by measuring the decline of the drug concentration in saliva (Welch et al., 1975).

The clinical application of the procedure indicated that a group of epileptic patients ($n = 10$) treated daily with anticonvulsant drugs for more than 2 months had a salivary antipyrine half-life (mean $\pm$ S.E.) of 4.2 hours $\pm$ 0.13 compared with 12.6 hours $\pm$ 0.95 in a group of normal volunteers ($n = 10$). Thus, the use of saliva instead of plasma for estimating the biological half-life of antipyrine is a convenient, rapid and sensitive procedure for evaluating the relative function of the drug-metabolizing system in humans. The half-lives of several drugs, including antipyrine, aminopyrine, phenacetin, digoxin, lithium, sulfonamides, barbiturates, theophylline and salicylates have been reported to be similar in plasma and saliva of humans; concentrations of some of these drugs were higher in plasma than in saliva. Elimination rates of heroin may differ in plasma and in saliva (Gorodetzky and Kullberg, 1974). Most assays of drug concentration in plasma measure the total (free + protein-bound) concentration present and fail to distinguish between the free and bound portions. Assuming that a compound enters saliva by passive diffusion, the concentration in saliva comprises only the free form of the drug. Apparent volumes of distribution of drugs, based on concentrations in plasma and saliva, should differ by the extent to which each drug is bound to plasma proteins. The greater the plasma protein binding, the lower the apparent volume of distribution in plasma compared with saliva.

The plasma antipyrine half-life (mean $\pm$ S.E.) in humans ($n=12$) is 12.7 hours $\pm$ 0.8 compared with 3.2 hours $\pm$ 0.28 in dogs ($n=6$). The salivary half-life of antipyrine (mean $\pm$ S.E.) in four male and four female rats was 101.8 min $\pm$ 8.3 and 146.3 min $\pm$ 8.2, respectively. The 45 per cent longer half-life of antipyrine in female rats is in agreement with the known ability of the male of this species to metabolize drugs faster than the female. Plasma antipyrine half-lives exhibited an inverse relationship to hepatic microsomal aniline hydroxylase and ethylmorphine N-demethylase activities in healthy mongrel dogs. However, no close correlation occurred between plasma antipyrine half-life and hepatic microsomal P-450 content, cytochrome c reductase activity or NADPH oxidase activity (Vesell et al., 1973). In dogs retested at 21 days, plasma antipyrine half-life was a highly reproducible value in each animal. However, at shorter time intervals the dose of antipyrine used (75 mg/kg, I.V.) probably induced hepatic microsomal drug metabolism, since retesting 10 days after the initial dose disclosed shortening of the plasma antipyrine half-life in each animal. Vesell and co-workers (1973) concluded that under certain conditions plasma antipyrine half-lives may be useful indices of rates of hepatic metabolism of several compounds chemically unrelated to antipyrine.

The plasma antipyrine half-lives (hours) in normal humans, dogs, rabbits and male and female rats are 12.7, 3.2, 1.1, 1.7 and 2.4, respectively. Interspecies variations in the rate of hepatic metabolism of antipyrine could be related to the increased liver mass relative to the total body weight of the smaller animals or to the blood flow rate to the liver.

The utility of biological half-life and clearance rate as indices of intrinsic hepatic drug elimination is highly dependent upon the pharmacokinetic characteristics of a particular drug (Perrier and Gibaldi, 1974). For drugs which confer the pharmacokinetic characteristics of a single compartment model on the body, both half-life and clearance serve as meaningful measures of hepatic elimination. A large number of drugs, however, confer on the body the characteristics of a multicompartment system rather than a simple one-compartment system. For this class of drugs the body does not behave as a single kinetically "homogeneous" compartment, but rather as two or more such compartments. For a drug which confers multicompartment characteristics on the body, biological half-life becomes a function not only of elimination but also of distribution. Hence its value as an index of hepatic elimination for this class of drugs becomes very questionable. Clearance, on the other hand, is a direct measure of hepatic elimination regardless of the number of compartments conferred upon the body by a drug, provided that the liver is part of the central compartment. For drugs subject to first-pass metabolism (Table 4–7), in

Table 4–7 DRUGS FOR WHICH FIRST-PASS
HEPATIC METABOLISM IS SUSPECTED

Propranolol	Diazepam
Guanethidine	Reserpine
Lidocaine	Naloxone
Nortriptyline	Meperidine
Imipramine	Phenacetin
Dopamine	Griseofulvin
Oxyphenbutazone	

which the liver becomes a compartment distinct from the central compartment, the applicability of clearance as an index of hepatic elimination becomes considerably more limited. After the intravenous administration of a drug that is subject to first-pass metabolism on oral administration, the reliability of body clearance as an index of hepatic elimination becomes less meaningful as the potential for first-pass metabolism increases. After oral drug administration, however, in which case the drug must pass through the liver prior to entering the systemic circulation, body clearance appears to reflect directly intrinsic metabolic activity regardless of the extent of first-pass metabolism. Irrespective of the route of drug administration, half-life serves as a poor index of hepatic elimination for drugs subject to significant first-pass metabolism.

The effect(s) of fever on drug disposition is (are) very interesting, but it is unclear at the present time whether the extent of distribution is changed or elimination (biotransformation and excretion) processes are altered. Even mild to moderate febrile reactions lead to significant alterations in hepatic clearance of sodium sulfobromophthalein (BSP), by producing increased reflux from the liver to the plasma and decreased relative hepatic storage capacity (Blaschke et al., 1973). Quinine disposition was studied in five subjects prior to and during an experimentally induced infection of falciparum malaria (Trenholme et al., 1976). The ratio of unmetabolized quinine (QB) to quinine plus quinine metabolites (QMPA) in plasma was interpreted as a measure of the extent of biotransformation of quinine. In all individuals, plasma levels of unmetabolized quinine and QB/QMPA ratios were increased during malaria, suggesting impaired hepatic metabolism of quinine. Increased plasma levels of quinine were attributed to a relative decrease in tissue distribution during the infection. The changes observed during malaria were not the result of altered renal excretion of quinine. The mean (plasma) half-life values of quinine before and during malaria were not significantly different. During the initial period of acute falciparum infections, when fever and other manifestations of the disease are most intense, higher plasma quinine levels and increased symptoms of cinchonism have been observed (Brooks et al., 1969; Powell and McNamara, 1972).

REFERENCES

Adamson, R. H. (1967): Drug metabolism in marine vertebrates. *Fed. Proc.*, 26:1047–1055.
Alary, J. G., Guay, P., and Brodeur, J. (1971): Effect of phenobarbital pretreatment on the metabolism of DDT in the rat and the bovine. *Toxicol. appl. Pharmacol.*, 18:457–468.

Alvin, J., McHorse, T., Hoyumpa, A., Bush, T. M., and Schenker, S. (1975): The effect of liver disease in man on the disposition of phenobarbital. *J. Pharmacol. exp. Ther.*, *192*:224–235.

Axelrod, J. (1954): Studies on sympathomimetic amines. II. The biotransformation and physiological disposition of *d*-amphetamine. *d*-p-hydroxyamphetamine and *d*-methamphetamine. *J. Pharmacol. Exp. Ther.*, *110*:315–326.

Baggot, J. D., and Davis, L. E. (1973): A comparative study of the pharmacokinetics of amphetamine. *Res. vet. Sci.*, *14*:207–215.

Black, M., and Billing, B. (1969): Hepatic bilirubin UDP-glucuronyl transferase activity in liver disease and Gilbert's syndrome. *New Engl. J. Med.*, *280*:1266–1271.

Blaschke, T. F., Elin, R. J., Berk, P. D., Song, C. S., and Wolff, S. M. (1973): Effect of induced fever on sulfobromophthalein kinetics in man. *Ann. intern. Med.*, *78*:221–226.

Branch, R. A., Shand, D. G., Wilkinson, G. R., and Nies. A. S. (1973): The reduction of lidocaine clearance by *dl*-propranolol:an example of hemodynamic drug interaction. *J. Pharmacol. exp. Ther.*, *184*:515–519.

Bridges, J. W., Kibby, M. R., Walker, S. R., and Williams. R. T. (1968): Species differences in the metabolism of sulphadimethoxine. *Biochem. J.*, *109*:851–856.

Brodie, B. B., and Axelrod, J. (1948): The fate of acetanilide in man. *J. Pharmacol. exp. Ther.*, *94*:29–38.

Brodie, B. B., and Axelrod, J. (1949): The fate of acetophenetidin (Phenacetin) in man and methods for the estimation of acetophenetidin and its metabolites in biological material. *J. Pharmacol. exp. Ther.* *97*:58–67.

Brodie, B. B., and Axelrod, J. (1950): The fate of antipyrine in man. *J. Pharmacol. exp. Ther.*, *98*:97–104.

Brodie, B. B., and Maickel, R. P. (1962): Comparative biochemistry of drug metabolism. *In* B. B. Brodie and E. G. Erdös (eds.): *Metabolic Factors Controlling Duration of Drug Action.* Proceedings of the First International Pharmacological Meeting. Vol. 6, Oxford, Pergamon Press, pp. 299–324.

Brodie, B. B., Gillette, J. R., and LaDu, B. N. (1958): Enzymatic metabolism of drugs and other foreign compounds. *Ann. Rev. Biochem.*, *27*:427–454.

Brooks, M. H., Malloy, J. P., Bartelloni, P. J., Sheehy, T. W., and Barry, K. G. (1969): Quinine, pyrimethamine, and sulforthodimethoxine: Clinical response, plasma levels, and urinary excretion during the initial attack of naturally acquired falciparum malaria. *Clin. Pharmacol. Ther.*, *10*:85–91.

Brownlee, G., and Williams, G. W. (1963): Potentiation of amphetamine and pethidine by monoamine oxidase inhibitors. *Lancet, 1*(7282):669.

Conney, A. H. (1967): Pharmacological implications of microsomal enzyme induction. *Pharmacol. Rev.*, *19*:317–366.

Conney, A. H., and Burns, J. J. (1972): Metabolic interactions among environmental chemicals and drugs. *Science, 178*:576–586.

Conney, A. H., Schneidman, K., Jacobson, M., and Kuntzman, R. (1965): Drug-induced changes in steroid metabolism. *Ann. N.Y. Acad. Sci., 123*:98–109.

Conney, A. H., Welch, R. M., Kuntzman, R., and Burns, J. J. (1967): Effects of pesticides on drug and steroid metabolism (commentary). *Clin. Pharmacol. Ther.*, *8*:2–10.

Cooper, J. R., Bloom, F. E., and Roth, R. H. (1970): *The Biochemical Basis of Neuropharmacology.* New York, Oxford University Press, pp. 137–139.

Cucinell, S. A., Conney, A. H., Sansur, M., and Burns, J. J. (1965): Drug interactions in man. I. Lowering effects of phenobarbital on plasma levels of bishydroxycoumarin (Dicumarol) and diphenylhydantoin (Dilantin). *Clin. Pharmacol. Ther.*, *6*:420–429.

Davies, D. S., Gigon, P. L., and Gillette, J. R. (1969): Species and sex differences in electron transport systems in liver microsomes and their relationship to ethylmorphine demethylation. *Life Sci.*, *8*:85–91.

Drayer, D., Reidenberg, M. M., and Sevy, R. W. (1974): N-acetyl procainamide: An active metabolite of procainamide. *Proc. Soc. Exp. Biol. Med.*, *146*:358–363.

Dreyfuss, J., Ross, J. J., and Schreiber, E. C. (1971): Absorption, excretion, and biotransformation of procainamide-^{14}C in the dog and rhesus monkey. *Arzneim. Forsch., 21*:948–951.

Dring, L. G., Smith, R. L., and Williams, R. T. (1970): The metabolic fate of amphetamine in man and other species. *Biochem. J., 116*:425–435.

Dutton, G. J. (1966): The biosynthesis of glucuronides. *In* G. J. Dutton (ed.): *Glucuronic Acid, Free and Combined. Chemistry, Biochemistry, Pharmacology and Medicine.* New York, Academic Press, pp. 185–299.

Ellison, T., Gutzait, L., and Van Loon, E. J. (1966): The comparative metabolism of *d*-amphetamine -^{14}C in the rat, dog and monkey. *J. Pharmacol. exp. Ther., 152:* 383–387.

Elson, J., Strong, J. M., Lee, W. -K., and Atkinson, A. J., Jr. (1975): Antiarrhythmic potency of N-acetylprocainamide. *Clin. Pharmacol. Ther., 17*:134–140.

Evans, G. H., Nies, A. S., and Shand, D. G. (1973): The disposition of propranolol. III. Decreased half-life and volume of distribution as a result of plasma binding in man, monkey, dog and rat. *J. Pharmacol. exp. Ther., 186*:114–122.

Faraj, B. A., Israili, Z. H., Perel, J. M., Jenkins, M. L., Holtzman, S. G., Cucinell, S. A., and Dayton, P. G. (1974): Metabolism and disposition of methylphenidate-^{14}C: studies in man and animals. *J. Pharmacol. exp. Ther., 191*:535–547.

Fouts, J. R. (1961): The metabolism of drugs by subfractions of hepatic microsomes. *Biochem. biophys. res. Comm., 6*:373–378.

Friedman, P. J., and Cooper, J. R. (1960): The role of alcohol dehydrogenase in the metabolism of chloral hydrate. *J. Pharmacol. exp. Ther., 129*:373–376.

Galeazzi, R. L., Sheiner, L. B., Lockwood, T., and Benet, L. Z. (1976): The renal elimination of procainamide. *Clin. Pharmacol. Ther., 19*:55–62.

Garrett, E. R., and Lambert, H. J. (1973): Pharmacokinetics of trichloroethanol and metabolites and interconversions among variously referenced pharmacokinetic parameters. *J. pharm. Sci., 62*:550–572.

Giardina, E.-G. V., Dreyfuss, J., Bigger, J. T., Jr., Shaw, J. M., and Schreiber, E. C. (1976): Metabolism of procainamide in normal and cardiac subjects. *Clin. Pharmacol. Ther., 19*:339–351.

Gillette, J. R. (1963): Metabolism of drugs and other foreign compounds by enzymatic mechanisms. *Rec. Progr. Drug Res., 6*:13–73.

Gillette, J. R. (1966): Biochemistry of drug oxidation and reduction by enzymes in hepatic endoplasmic reticulum. *Adv. Pharmacol., 4*:219–261.

Gillette, J. R. (1971*a*): Techniques for studying drug metabolism *in vitro. In* B. N. LaDu, H. G. Mandel and E. L. Way (eds.): *Fundamentals of Drug Metabolism and Drug Disposition.* Baltimore, Williams & Wilkins, pp. 400–418.

Gillette, J. R. (1971*b*): Factors affecting drug metabolism. *Ann. N.Y. Acad. Sci., 179*:43–66.

Goodman, L. S.,and Gilman, A. (1975): *The Pharmacological Basis of Therapeutics.* 5th Ed. New York, Macmillan.

Gorodetzky, C. W., and Kullberg, M. P. (1974): Validity of screening methods for drugs of abuse in biological fluids. II. Heroin in plasma and saliva. *Clin. Pharmacol. Ther., 15*:579–587.

Govier, W. C. (1965): Reticuloendothelial cells as the site of sulfanilamide acetylation in the rabbit. *J. Pharmacol. exp. Ther., 150*:305–308.

Hayaishi, O. (1962): History and scope. *In* O. Hayaishi (ed.): *Oxygenases.* New York, Academic Press, pp. 1–29.

Held, H., and Oldershausen, H. F. V. (1969): Zur pharmakokinetik von meprobamat bei chronischen hepatopathien und arzneimittelsucht. *Klin. Wschr., 47*:78–80.

Hofstee, B. H. J. (1956): Graphical analysis of single enzyme systems. *Enzymologia, 17*:273–278.

Horwitz, D., Lovenberg, W., Engleman, K., and Sjoerdsma, A. (1964): Monoamine oxidase inhibitors, tyramine, and cheese. *J.A.M.A., 188*:1108–1110.

Huffman, D. H., Shoeman, D. W., and Azarnoff, D. L. (1974): Correlation of the plasma elimination of antipyrine and the appearance of 4-hydroxyantipyrine in the urine. *Biochem. Pharmacol., 23*:197–201.

Hvidberg, E. F., Andreasen, P. B., and Ranek, L. (1974): Plasma half-life of phenylbutazone in patients with impaired liver function. *Clin. Pharmacol. Ther., 15*:171–177.

Isselbacher, K. J., Chrabas, M. F., and Quinn, R. C. (1962): The solubilization and partial purification of a glucuronyl transferase from rabbit liver microsomes. *J. Biol. Chem., 237*:3033–3036.

Keenaghan, J. B., and Boyes, R. N. (1972): The tissue distribution, metabolism and excretion of lidocaine in rats, guinea pigs, dogs and man. *J. Pharmacol. exp. Ther., 180*:454–463.

Klotz, U., McHorse, T. S., Wilkinson, G. R., and Schenker, S. (1974): The effect of cirrhosis on the disposition and elimination of meperidine in man. *Clin. Pharmacol. Ther., 16*:667–679.

Kolmodin, B., Azarnoff, D. L., and Sjoqvist, F. (1969): Effect of environmental factors on drug metabolism: decreased plasma half-life of antipyrine in workers exposed to chlorinated hydrocarbon insecticides. *Clin. Pharmacol. Ther., 10*:638–642.

Kunin, C. M., Glazko, A. J., and Finland, M. (1959): Persistence of antibiotics in blood of patients with acute renal failure. II. Chloramphenicol and its metabolic products in blood of patients with severe renal disease or hepatic cirrhosis. *J. clin. Invest., 38*:1498–1508.

Levi, A. J., Sherlock, S., and Walker, D. (1968): Phenylbutazone isoniazid metabolism in patients with liver disease in relation to previous drug therapy. *Lancet, 1*:1275–1279.

Lineweaver, H., and Burk, D. (1934): The determination of enzyme dissociation constants. *J. Am. chem. Soc., 56*:658–666.

Loomis, T. A. (1968): *Essentials of Toxicology.* Philadelphia, Lea & Febiger.

Mackay, F. J., and Cooper, J. R. (1962): A study on the hypnotic activity of chloral hydrate. *J. Pharmacol. exp. Ther., 135*:271–274.

Mason, H. S. (1957): Mechanisms of oxygen metabolism. *Science, 125*:1185–1188.

Mawer, G. E., Miller, N. E., and Turnberg, L. A. (1972): Metabolism of amylobarbitone in patients with chronic liver disease. *Brit. J. Pharmacol., 44*:549–560.

Muting, D., and Reikowski, H. (1965): Protein metabolism in liver disease. *In* H. Popper and F. Schaffner (eds.): *Progress in Liver Diseases.* Vol. II. New York, Grune & Stratton, pp. 84–94.

Nose, Y., and Lipmann, F. (1958): Separation of steroid sulfokinases. *J. Biol. Chem., 233*:1348–1351.

Omura, T., and Sato, R. (1964a): The carbon monoxide-binding pigment of liver microsomes. I. Evidence for its haemoprotein nature. *J. Biol. Chem., 239*:2370–2378.

Omura, T., and Sato, R. (1964b): The carbon monoxide-binding pigment of liver microsomes. II. Solubilization, purification and properties. *J. Biol. Chem., 239*:2379–2385.

Orrenius, S. (1971): Molecular aspects of drug metabolism. *Acta Pharmacol. Toxical., 29*: (Suppl. 3): 191–202.

Parke, D. V. (1968): *The Biochemistry of Foreign Compounds.* Oxford, Pergamon Press, pp. 117–136.

Perrier, D., and Gibaldi, M. (1974): Clearance and biologic half-life as indices of intrinsic hepatic metabolism. *J. Pharmacol. exp. Ther., 191*:17–24.

Powell, R. D., and McNamara, J. V. (1972): Quinine: Side effects and plasma levels. *Proc. Helminth. Soc. Wash., 39*:331–338.

Prescott, L. F., Adjepon-Yamoah, K. K., and Roberts, E. (1973): Rapid gas-liquid chromatographic estimation of antipyrine in plasma. *J. Pharm. Pharmacol., 25*:205–207.

Remmer, H. (1972): Induction of drug metabolizing enzyme system in the liver. *Europ. J. clin. Pharmacol., 5*:116–136.

Robbins, P. W., and Lipmann, F. (1957): Isolation and identification of active sulfate. *J. Biol. Chem., 229*:837–851.

Rosso, R., Donelli, M. G., Francki, G., and Garattini, S. (1971): Impairment of drug metabolism in tumor-bearing animals. *Europ. J. Cancer, 7*:565–577.

Rumack, B. H., Holtzman, J., and Chase, H. P. (1973): Hepatic drug metabolism and protein malnutrition. *J. Pharmacol. exp. Ther., 186*:441–446.

Scatchard, G. (1949): The attractions of proteins for small molecules and ions. *Ann. N. Y. Acad. Sci.*, *51*:660–692.

Scheline, R. R. (1968): Drug metabolism by intestinal microorganisms. *J. pharm. Sci.*, *57*:2021–2037.

Schoene, B., Fleischmann, R. A., Remmer, H., and Oldershausen, H. F. V. (1972): Determination of drug metabolizing enzymes in needle biopsies of human liver. *Europ. J. clin. Pharmacol.*, *4*:65–73.

Sjoqvist, F. (1965): Psychotropic drugs. II. Interaction between monoamine oxidase (MAO) inhibitors and other substances. *Proc. Roy. Soc. Med.*, *58*:967–978.

Smith, J. N. (1968): Comparative metabolism of xenobiotics. *In* O. Lowenstein (ed.): *Advances in Comparative Physiology and Biochemistry*. Vol. 3. New York, Academic Press, pp. 173–232.

Smith, R. L., and Williams, R. T. (1966): Implications of the conjugation of drugs and other exogenous compounds. *In* G. J. Dutton (ed.): *Glucuronic Acid, Free and Combined. Chemistry, Biochemistry, Pharmacology and Medicine*. New York, Academic Press, pp. 457–491.

Soberman, R., Brodie, B. B., Levy, B. B., Axelrod, J., Hollander, V., and Steele, J. M. (1949): The use of antipyrine in the measurement of total body water in man. *J. Biol. Chem.*, *179*:31–42.

Stekol, J. A. (1936): Comparative studies in the sulfur metabolism of the dog and pig. *J. Biol. Chem.*, *113*:675–682.

Stripp, B., Greene, F. E., and Gillette, J. R. (1969): Disulfiram impairment of drug metabolism by rat liver microsomes. *J. Pharmacol. exp. Ther.*, *170*:347–354.

Tavernor, W. D. (1971): Muscle relaxants. *In* L. R. Soma (ed.): *Textbook of Veterinary Anesthesia*. Baltimore, Williams & Wilkins.

Thomson, P. D., Melmon, K. L., Richardson, J. A., Cohn, K., Steinbrunn, W., Cudihee, R., and Rowland, M. (1973): Lidocaine pharmacokinetics in advanced heart failure, liver disease, and renal failure in humans. *Ann. intern. Med.*, *78*:499–508.

Trenholme, G. M., Williams, R. L., Rieckmann, K. H., Frischer, H., and Carson, P. E. (1976): Quinine disposition during malaria and during induced fever. *Clin. Pharmacol. Ther.*, *19*:459–467.

Tygstrup, N. (1964): The galactose elimination capacity in control subjects and in patients with cirrhosis of the liver. *Acta med. Scand.*, *175*:281–289.

Vesell, E. S., Passananti, G. T., and Greene, F. E. (1970): Impairment of drug metabolism in man by allopurinol and nortriptyline. *N. Engl. J. Med.*, *283*:1484–1488.

Vesell, E. S., Passananti, G. T., and Lee, C. H. (1971): Impairment of drug metabolism by disulfiram in man. *Clin. Pharmacol. Ther.*, *12*:785–792.

Vesell, E. S., Lee, C. J., Passananti, G. T., and Shively, C. A. (1973): Relationship between plasma antipyrine half-lives and hepatic microsomal drug metabolism in dogs. *Pharmacology*, *10*:317–328.

Vesell, E. S., Passananti, G. T., Glenwright, P. A., and Dvorchik, B. H. (1975a): Studies on the disposition of antipyrine, aminopyrine, and phenacetin using plasma, saliva, and urine. *Clin. Pharmacol. Ther.*, *18*:259–272.

Vesell, E. S., Passananti, G. T., Viau, J. P., Epps, J. E., and DiCarlo, F. J. (1972): Effects of chronic prazepam administration on drug metabolism in man and rat. *Pharmacology*, *7*:192–206.

Vesell, E. S., Shapiro, J. R., Passananti, G. T., Jorgensen, H., and Shively, C. A. (1975b): Altered plasma half-lives of antipyrine, propylthiouracil, and methimazole in thyroid dysfunction. *Clin. Pharmacol. Ther.*, *17*:48–56.

Walle, T., and Gaffney, T. E. (1972): Propranolol metabolism in man and dog: mass spectrometric identification of six new metabolites. *J. Pharmacol. exp. Ther.*, *182*:83–92.

Welch, R. M., DeAngelis, R. L., Wingfield, M., and Farmer, T. W. (1975): Elimination of antipyrine from saliva as a measure of metabolism in man. *Clin. Pharmacol. Ther.*, *18*:249–258.

Welch, R. M., Harrison, Y. E., and Burns, J. J. (1967): Implications of enzyme induction in drug toxicity studies. *Toxicol. appl. Pharmacol.*, *10*:340–351.

Wilkinson, G. R. (1975): Pharmacokinetics of drug disposition: hemodynamic considerations. *Ann. Rev. Pharmacol., 15*:11–27.

Williams, R. T. (1959): *Detoxication Mechanisms.* 2nd Ed. London, Chapman and Hall.

Williams, R. T. (1967*a*): Comparative patterns of drug metabolism. *Fed. Proc., 26*:1029–1039.

Williams, R. T. (1967*b*): The biogenesis of conjugation and detoxication products. *In* P. Bernfeld (ed.): 2nd Ed. *Biogenesis of Natural Compounds.* Oxford, Pergamon Press, pp. 590–639.

Williams, R. T. (1971): Species variations in drug biotransformations. *In* B. N. LaDu, H. G. Mandel and E. L. Way (eds.): *Fundamentals of Drug Metabolism and Drug Disposition.* Baltimore, Williams & Wilkins, pp. 187–205.

Williams, R. T. (1972): Toxicologic implications of biotransformation by intestinal microflora. *Toxicol. appl. Pharmacol., 23*:769–781.

Woolf, B. (1932): Cited in J. B. S. Haldane and L. G. Stern: *Allgemeine Chemic der Enzyme.* Dresen, Steinkopff Verlag, p. 119.

5
Mechanisms of Drug Excretion

INTRODUCTION

Drugs and other foreign chemical compounds are eliminated from the body by a combination of biotransformation and excretion processes. Although the kidneys are the principal organ of excretion, the liver, salivary glands, mammary glands (in lactating animals) and sweat glands constitute nonrenal routes of excretion. Volatile agents diffuse from the blood into pulmonary alveolar spaces and are exhaled.

The degree of lipid-solubility and extent of ionization in biological fluids are the main factors that determine the proportion of the therapeutic dose of any drug eliminated by excretion. Polar drugs and the majority of drug metabolites are excreted in the urine. Although most excretion processes are passive (nonionic diffusion) in nature, some are carrier-mediated and active. Excretion usually obeys first-order kinetics, but when drug levels in plasma exceed the capacity of specialized transport processes (e.g., carrier-mediated excretion of some drugs and many metabolites into urine and bile), the excretion kinetics become zero-order.

Renal impairment, in particular reduced glomerular filtration rate, delays excretion of drugs that are eliminated predominantly unchanged in urine. Some consequences of reduced renal function are an increase in half-life of these drugs, a prolonged duration of action, and a need to lengthen dosage interval so that excessive drug accumulation and toxicity will be avoided. Uremia may cause a de-

113

crease in drug binding to plasma proteins and a reduction in the rates of some biotransformation pathways. Administration of the usual dose will produce an increased pharmacological response. The observation that uremic animals appear "more sensitive" to the action of some drugs may be attributed to alterations in disposition (distribution and elimination) of the drugs.

RENAL EXCRETION

Physiological Basis of Kidney Function

The role of the kidneys is primarily to regulate the volume and composition of the internal fluid environment; their excretory function is incidental to their regulatory function (Pitts, 1968). The most important feature of the mammalian renal system is its highly developed anatomical arrangement in which renal cells are interposed between blood and tubular fluid. The kidneys receive the greatest blood flow, in proportion to weight, of any organ of the body. At rest, renal blood flow amounts to 20 to 25 per cent of cardiac output; the kidneys constitute only 0.4 per cent of body weight. Regulation of the internal environment is a composite of four processes:

1. *Ultrafiltration of blood plasma at the glomerulus.* The filtration process is passive and nonselective. Glomerular filtration of solutes is limited by the size and shape of each solute present in plasma. Albumin molecules, which have a diameter slightly less than that of the pores in the glomerular capillary walls, are largely sieved (restrained) by the combined effects of steric hindrance, viscous drag and electrical hindrance. It is virtually impossible to determine the extent to which protein binding impedes the glomerular filtration of a drug.

2. *Secretion by the tubules of certain substances from blood into the tubular lumen for addition to urine.* Three types of secretory mechanisms are involved in the transport of materials from peritubular fluid to tubular lumen: (*a*) Active secretory mechanisms, which exhibit an absolute limitation of transport capacity. Organic acids and organic bases are secreted by distinct mechanisms, both of which are localized in the proximal tubule. (*b*) Hydrogen ions are transported by an active mechanism which exhibits gradient- and perhaps time-limited transport capacity. This mechanism is present throughout the length of the nephron but is diversely specialized in its several parts. (*c*) Passive secretory mechanisms, which involve diffusion of materials down concentration gradients or electrical poten-

tial gradients. Weak organic bases with pK_a values between 6.85 and 9.35 and certain acidic drugs (e.g., salicylic acid and phenobarbital) diffuse passively into and become trapped (by ionization) in acidic and alkaline tubular fluid, respectively. Passive secretion of weak organic electrolytes occurs in all regions of the tubule but is most evident in those in which the highest hydrogen ion gradients are established—namely, in its terminal portions. Most of the filtered potassium ion is reabsorbed in the proximal tubule. The potassium that is excreted in urine apparently is added to tubular fluid in the distal nephron. The secretion of potassium ions is passive and occurs down a potential gradient established by the active reabsorption of sodium ions.

3. *Selective reabsorption by the tubules of materials required in maintaining the internal environment* (e.g., water, sodium, potassium, chloride and bicarbonate ions, glucose, phosphate, sulfate, amino acids and certain organic acids of the Krebs cycle). The reabsorptive mechanism for glucose has the characteristics of an active system with limited capacity (i.e., the tubular transport system has a maximal rate, T_m). Under normal conditions, all the glucose in the glomerular filtrate is actively reabsorbed in the proximal convoluted tubule. When the plasma concentration of glucose exceeds some critical level, termed the "renal plasma threshold," glucose appears in the urine. Glycosuria in association with polyuria, polydipsia and polyphagia is characteristic of diabetes mellitus. The major ions of extracellular fluid, namely, sodium, chloride and bicarbonate, are reabsorbed by active mechanisms that exhibit gradient- and time-limited transport capacity. Water, chloride and urea are reabsorbed passively along gradients of osmotic activity, electrical potential and concentration, respectively. The translocation of ions and water in a nephron is shown diagrammatically in Figure 5–1.

At this point it may be appropriate to state that three basic factors are involved in converting the isotonic glomerular filtrate to a concentrated urine: (*a*) active reabsorption of the major urinary solutes, particularly sodium and its attendant anions; (*b*) the action of antidiuretic hormone (ADH) in controlling permeability of the distal convoluted tubule and collecting ducts to water; (*c*) a hypertonic medullary interstitium, which is maintained by the activities of the loop of Henle. The principal stimulus for release of ADH from the neurohypophysis is the effective osmolarity of extracellular fluid.

4. *Precise regulation of the internal fluid environmental pH* (7.35 to 7.45) is attained through the operation of both chemical and physiological (respiratory system and kidneys) buffering mechanisms. The kidneys eliminate the fixed (nonvolatile) acid and basic end-products

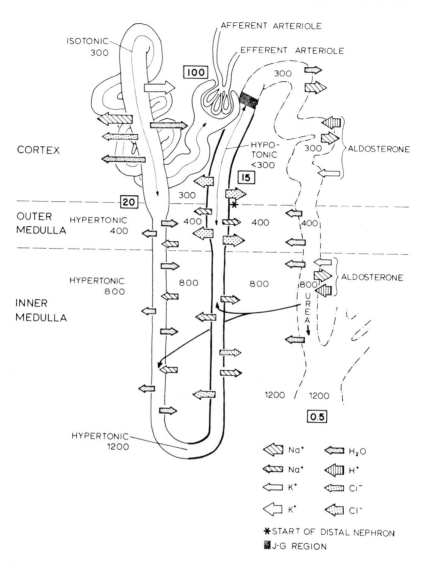

Figure 5–1 Schematic representation of mammalian nephron showing sites and processes of ion (Na+, K+, Cl−, H+) and water transport. The various segments of the nephron have different transport characteristics. Broad arrows indicate active transport; narrow ones represent passive diffusion. Membrane permeability to water varies with the segment of the nephron. The proximal tubular epithelium and descending limb of Henle's loop are highly permeable to osmotic flow of water, whereas the thin and medullary thick portions of the ascending limb of Henle's loop are completely impermeable. Membrane permeability to water is low in the diluting segment and variable in the other segments (− · − · −) of the distal nephron, depending on the level of antidiuretic hormone. Concentrations of tubular urine and peritubular fluid shown are for the human and expressed in mOsm/liter; boxed numerals are the estimated per cent of glomerular filtrate remaining within the nephron at various segments.

BASIC ION EXCHANGE MECHANISM

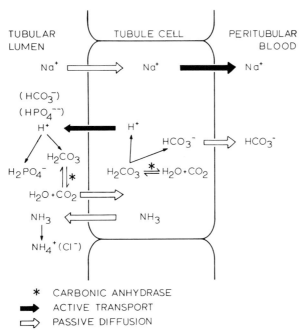

Figure 5–2   General scheme showing the exchange of hydrogen ions, which were derived from carbonic acid, for sodium ions of tubular fluid. This exchange takes place in the reabsorption of bicarbonate and in urinary excretion of titratable acid and ammonia. Carbonic anhydrase is present in renal tubule cells and within the lumen of proximal tubular segment, where it is attached to the brush border of cells.

of metabolism and regulate precisely the concentration of bicarbonate ion in body fluids. The basic ion exchange mechanism of a proximal tubule cell is shown schematically in Figure 5–2.

Renal Excretion of Drugs

Renal excretion is the principal process of elimination for drugs that have limited lipid-solubility or are predominantly ionized within the physiological range of pH. Drugs that are excreted mainly unchanged in urine include many antibiotics (e.g., penicillins, cephalosporins, aminoglycosides, oxytetracycline), nondepolarizing (competitive) neuromuscular blocking agents (e.g., d-tubocurarine and gallamine triethiodide), most diuretics (with the notable exception of ethacrynic acid) and digoxin. Renal excretion of drugs is complex and involves the processes of glomerular filtration, carrier-mediated excretion in the proximal convoluted tubules and passive reabsorption, by diffusion, in the distal portion of the nephron.

Drug molecules that are free in the blood plasma will pass through the porous glomerular capillary membrane into the tubular lumen. The amount of drug entering the tubular lumen by filtration is dependent on its degree of binding to plasma proteins and the glomerular filtration rate. Since the drug concentration increases progressively as water is reabsorbed from the glomerular filtrate, a concentration gradient favoring drug reabsorption is established as the filtrate moves along the nephron. The tubular epithelium is permeable only to lipid-soluble drug molecules. Since lipid-solubility is a feature of only the nonionized form of weak organic electrolytes, the extent of their reabsorption is determined by the pH of tubular fluid and the pK_a value of the drug (Milne et al., 1958). Foreign compounds that have low lipid-solubility or are highly ionized will be excreted, whereas compounds of high lipid-solubility may be reabsorbed from tubular fluid into the blood. The normal urinary pH of carnivores, such as the dog and cat, is acidic (5.5 to 7.0), while that of horses, cattle and sheep (herbivorous species) is alkaline (7.0 to 8.0). In any species, however, urinary pH is dependent on the diet. Animal protein and grains with high protein content tend to produce an acid urine, whereas vegetables and grasses (including hay) generally result in an alkaline urine. Omnivores, such as swine, may excrete an acid or alkaline urine. In the human, the urine is usually acid but can vary over a wide pH range (5.0 to 7.5). Suckling and milk-fed animals generally produce an acid urine even if in adult life they characteristically excrete an alkaline urine. The extent to which urinary pH influences the rate of renal excretion of an organic electrolyte depends largely upon the concentration and degree of ionization of the drug in tubular fluid. Tubular reabsorption by the process of nonionic diffusion is a feature of the renal handling of organic acids with pK_a values within the range 3.0 to 7.2 when the urine is acid, and of organic bases with pK_a values between 8.0 and 11.0 when the urine is alkaline. Although the excretion rate of several drugs may be altered by changing urinary pH, this technique will have little clinical application unless a significant fraction of the dose is excreted unchanged in the urine. Since wide species variations exist in the fate of lipid-soluble drugs, the relative proportions of any dose that are eliminated by excretion and biotransformation are species dependent. In humans and probably in dogs, alkalinization of the urine increases the excretion of salicylate (pK_a 3.0), sulfisoxazole (pK_a 5.0) and phenobarbital (pK_a 7.2), whereas urinary acidification hastens excretion (i.e., decreases the half-life) of amphetamine (pK_a 9.9). Induction of an alkaline diuresis may successfully combat intoxication caused by overdosage with a lipid-soluble weak organic acid.

The relationship between glomerular filtration rate and the clearance of a drug that is excreted mainly unchanged in urine and not transported into tubular fluid by a specialized process is influenced by plasma protein binding of the drug, the magnitude of distribution in body fluids and the extent of passive reabsorption from tubular fluid. When therapeutic doses are administered, the renal excretion mechanisms generally have the net effect of eliminating a constant fraction of the drug presented to the kidneys by the renal arterial blood — i.e., excretion is usually a first-order process.

Any pharmacologically active compound that lowers blood pressure or constricts renal arterioles will reduce the glomerular filtration rate (GFR). The effect of reduced GFR on renal excretion of a drug which is "secreted" by the renal tubules will be considerably less than that for drugs excreted by filtration alone. Certain drugs (e.g., penicillins, furosemide) and many drug metabolites, in particular conjugates (i.e., phase II metabolic products), are excreted into renal tubular fluid by carrier-mediated transport processes (Weiner and Mudge, 1964). Molecules diffuse from the peritubular capillary network which surrounds the proximal convoluted tubule into extracellular fluid. On entering a renal tubule cell membrane or having traversed the membrane, drug molecules combine with a transporting carrier substance, which is present in limited amount, and are released into the lumen of the tubule. Throughout its length, the proximal tubule is composed of a single layer of cuboidal or truncated pyramidal cells resting on an enveloping basal lamina. Some organic substances whose passage through renal epithelial cells is carrier-mediated are listed in Table

Table 5–1   DRUGS EXCRETED IN THE PROXIMAL PORTION OF THE RENAL TUBULE BY CARRIER-MEDIATED TRANSPORT PROCESSES

Acids	Bases
Penicillin G	Procainamide
Phenylbutazone	Mecamylamine
Probenecid	Dopamine
Salicylic acid	Quinine
Sulfisoxazole	Quaternary ammonium compounds
Acetazolamide	(e.g., tetraethylammonium)
Chlorothiazide	N-Methylnicotinamide
Furosemide	Trimethoprim
Para-aminohippurate	
Glucuronic acid conjugates	
Ethereal sulfates	

5–1. Although the tubular transport systems responsible for secretion of organic anions and cations are independent, both have similar characteristics and are located in the proximal region of the nephron. The tubular transport processes require an energy source and carrier substances, which are relatively nonspecific and handle either organic anions or cations. The transport system is susceptible to interference by metabolic or competitive inhibitors and rapidly removes certain foreign organic compounds (includes metabolites) from blood, but has a limited capacity. Above a certain plasma concentration of drug, the carrier-mediated system becomes saturated and transport proceeds at a maximal rate by apparent zero-order kinetics. Binding to plasma proteins does not hinder tubular excretion of drugs, presumably because the drug-albumin complex dissociates immediately upon removal of free drug from the plasma. The penicillin analogues cloxacillin and ampicillin are approximately 80 per cent and 20 per cent bound, respectively, to plasma albumin, are excreted by similar renal mechanisms and have the same half-life (1.2 hours) in cows. Conclusive evidence for tubular secretion of a drug must include data showing that the carrier-mediated process can be inhibited. Concurrent administration of either acidic or basic drugs that are substrates for carrier-mediated excretion processes will prolong persistence in the body of the less readily transported (secreted) compound. Probenecid and phenylbutazone, substrates for the organic acid system, reduce renal tubular excretion of penicillin and thereby decrease the rate of elimination (i.e., prolong the half-life) of the antibiotic (Kampmann et al., 1972). Even though some drugs enter tubular fluid by glomerular filtration and carrier-mediated excretion, their renal clearance may be low because they are substantially reabsorbed in the distal portion of the nephron. The handling of salicylate by renal mechanisms in dogs and cats exemplifies this point.

Renal Clearance

The renal clearance of a substance is defined as the volume of plasma completely cleared of that substance by the kidneys per unit time, and is expressed in milliliters per minute. The rate of glomerular filtration can be determined by measuring the renal clearance of substances that are freely filterable through glomerular capillaries, are neither secreted nor reabsorbed by the tubules and exert no effect on renal function (Smith, 1956). Compounds which meet these criteria are inulin, a polymeric carbohydrate with a molecular weight of 5200, and infused creatinine (in domestic animals but not in humans). The clearance of inulin, obtained from the relationship:

$$\text{Clearance}_{(\text{inulin})} = \frac{\text{Urinary concentration of inulin} \times \text{Urine flow rate}}{\text{Plasma concentration of inulin}}$$

Equation 5 • 1

accurately measures the rate of glomerular filtration in all mammalian species when the plasma inulin concentration is maintained relatively constant. It is essential that blood samples for inulin determination be obtained at the midpoint of each urine collection period. Another way of expressing Equation 5 · 1 is:

$$\text{Clearance (ml/min)} = \frac{\text{Excretion rate (mg/min)}}{\text{Plasma concentration (mg/ml)}}$$ **Equation 5 • 2**

The clearance of inulin is a measure of the volume of plasma filtered through the glomeruli each minute. The most common cause of reduction in the filtration rate is organic change in the renal vascular bed. A decrease in renal blood flow will reduce filtration rate and occurs in heart failure and as a side-effect of therapy with certain drugs (e.g., guanethidine). Although binding to plasma proteins reduces availability of a portion of the circulating drug for glomerular filtration, it may not exert a controlling effect on the overall rate of excretion.

The renal mechanisms for excretion of para-aminohippurate (PAH) and iodopyracet (Diodrast) include glomerular filtration and tubular secretion. These substances are excreted so efficiently at low plasma levels that essentially all of the substance is removed from the blood in a single passage through the kidney. It therefore follows that the total amount of such a substance excreted in the urine over a given time divided by its plasma concentration is an expression of renal plasma flow. The clearance of PAH at low plasma PAH concentrations (<5 mg/100 ml), obtained by applying Equation 5 · 1, serves as a measure of the effective renal plasma flow (ERPF). The extraction of PAH in a single passage through the kidney of the human being is, on an average, 90 per cent complete (Smith, 1951). In the dog, extraction of PAH is appreciably less complete, averaging 75 to 80 per cent. Renal clearance values of inulin, creatinine and either PAH or Diodrast in normal domestic animals are presented in Table 5–2. From a pharmacological viewpoint, the much lower value of the renal clearance of inulin in the horse and cow compared with that in the dog is the most important feature of the species variation in renal function.

Blood urea nitrogen (BUN) concentration and serum creatinine (SC) concentration can be regarded only as crude indices of renal function in dogs and cats (Finco and Duncan, 1976). Many nonrenal

Table 5–2 RENAL CLEARANCE VALUES IN ADULT ANIMALS OF DIFFERENT SPECIES

Species	Substance Cleared	Median Value (ml/min/kg) (range in parentheses)
Horse*	Inulin	1.66 (1.00–2.32)
	Creatinine	1.46 (1.02–1.90)
	Diodrast	6.91 (5.29–8.53)
	Urea	0.76 (0.56–0.96)
Cow†	Inulin	1.84 (1.30–2.20)
	Creatinine	1.68 (1.32–2.23)
	Diodrast	9.11 (5.82–12.60)
	Urea	0.84 (0.56–1.00)
Pig‡	Inulin	2.1 (1.8–2.5)
	Creatinine	2.2 (1.5–3.4)
	Para-aminohippurate	6.4 (5.2–8.4)
	Urea	1.2 (0.9–1.8)
Dog§	Inulin	3.77 (1.74–5.86)
	Creatinine	4.3 (2.2 –8.3)
	Para-aminohippurate	12.88 (6.30–21.18)

*Knudsen, E. (1959): *Acta vet. scand., 1*:52.
†Poulsen, E. (1957): *R. vet. agric. College Copenhagen*, Yearbook.
‡Gyrd-Hansen, N. (1968): *Acta vet. scand., 9*:183.
§Asheim, A., Persson, F., and Persson, S. (1961): *Acta physiol. scand., 51*:150.

factors influence the serum concentration of urea and creatinine. Renal excretion is quantitatively the most important process of urea elimination. Urea undergoes glomerular filtration and a portion is passively reabsorbed by the renal tubules. The amount of urea reabsorbed is related to the rate of passage of filtrate through the tubules.

In all mammalian species, creatinine is freely filtered through the glomerulus, appearing in glomerular filtrate in the same concentration as in plasma (Smith, 1951). Species differences exist with regard to tubular action on creatinine. In humans, creatinine is secreted by the tubules apparently by the same mechanism that transports PAH and other organic acids. For many years, the renal tubules of dogs, sheep and seals have been considered to be qualitatively different from those of rats, apes and humans, in that the former are unable to secrete creatinine. Evidence suggests that the difference may be quantitative rather than qualitative (Swanson and Hakim, 1962; O'Connell et al., 1962). The creatinine and inulin clearances of the dog and other species of domestic animals are the same, within limits of experimental error, under conventional free-flow conditions. Based on BUN and SC data from 111 azotemic dogs and cats, Finco and Duncan

(1976) concluded that single determinations of BUN or SC provide no basis for prognosis.

For clinical evaluation of renal function, clearances of the radioiodine compounds sodium ^{125}I-iothalamate (Glofil-125*) and sodium ^{131}I-iodohippurate (Hipputope†) given as a single intravenous injection may be satisfactory indices of renal function. The clearance is obtained from the product of the first-order overall elimination rate constant and the apparent volume of distribution of the agent, and is equal to the renal clearance when the agent is cleared from the body entirely by the kidneys. By measuring decline of ^{125}I-iothalamate and ^{131}I-iodohippurate from plasma after giving a single intravenous injection, clearances of the radioisotopes were obtained in normal beagles and cats (Table 5–3). A distinct advantage of this method is that infusion of the agents and collection of urine, for measurement purposes, are not necessary. The urine voided during the 48 hours after administering the radioisotopes must, however, be collected and disposed of in the proper manner. The single injection technique should provide a rapid means of assessing renal function to assist in the diagnosis of renal disease. Knowledge of the renal function status of an animal is required in designing dosage regimens of drugs with a narrow therapeutic index (such as cardiac glycosides, procainamide,

---

*Glofil-125, Abbott Laboratories, Radio-Pharmaceutical Products Division, North Chicago, Illinois.

†Hipputope, Squibb & Sons, E. R., Princeton, New Jersey.

Table 5–3 MEASUREMENT OF RENAL FUNCTION IN BEAGLE DOGS AND IN CATS BY DETERMINING CLEARANCE OF RADIOIODINE COMPOUNDS

Compound Cleared	Half-Life (min) Mean ± S.D.	Body Clearance (ml/kg/min) Mean ± S.D.	Renal Process Measured
Dogs (n = 11):			
[125]I-Iothalamate	36.1 ± 6.6	4.5 ± 2.0	Glomerular filtration rate (GFR)
[131]I-Iodohippurate	16.3 ± 3.0	12.9 ± 1.7	Effective renal plasma flow (ERPF)
Cats (n = 10)*			
[125]I-Iothalamate	33.6 ± 4.5	5.1 ± 1.5	GFR
[131]I-Iodohippurate	19.0 ± 4.6	14.1 ± 5.7	ERPF

*Data from Mercer, H. D. (1976): Personal communication.

[125]I-Iothalamate sodium (Glofil-125): Abbott Laboratories, Radio-Pharmaceuticals Division, North Chicago, Illinois.

[131]I-Iodohippurate (Hipputope): Squibb & Sons, E. R., Princeton, New Jersey.

aminoglycosides, cephalosporins, oxytetracycline) when renal impairment would lead to accumulation of drug to toxic levels unless the usual dosage regimen is modified. The increase in average amount of drug in the body will depend on severity of the renal failure and the contribution of the renal route to the total elimination of the drug.

Since creatinine appears to be eliminated from the body almost entirely by renal excretion, its (total) body clearance can be considered to represent renal clearance. The biological half-life of a drug (or compound such as creatinine) can be estimated from knowledge of its apparent volume of distribution and clearance value:

$$\text{Drug half-life} = \frac{0.693 \times \text{Volume of distribution}}{\text{Body clearance}} \qquad \textbf{Equation 5 • 3}$$

The creatinine clearance can be estimated by dividing the urinary creatinine excretion rate by the average concentration of serum creatinine (Equation 5 · 2). In patients with renal impairment, the serum creatinine concentration increases until a higher steady state is established. The time required to reach the higher steady state serum creatinine level after onset of renal failure is highly dependent upon the degree of renal insufficiency (Chiou and Hsu, 1975). The value of renal clearance only infrequently is the same as that of body clearance, as the majority of drugs are eliminated by a combination of excretion and biotransformation processes. Since creatinine is excreted almost entirely unchanged in the urine, its first-order elimination rate constant in patients with impaired renal function should be directly proportional to the fraction of normal renal function remaining in these patients. The biological half-life of creatinine in patients with impaired renal function can be estimated by the relationship:

$t_{1/2}$ (impaired renal function)

$$= \frac{t_{1/2} \text{ (normal)}}{\text{Fraction of normal renal function remaining}} \qquad \textbf{Equation 5 • 4}$$

The fraction of normal renal function remaining is most commonly estimated by the apparent creatinine clearance method (Tozer, 1974).

MECHANISMS OF ACTION OF DIURETICS

Diuretics are agents that increase the rate of urine formation. Most diuretics exert their action directly on the kidney and, with few exceptions, on tubular rather than glomerular function. These drugs provide symptomatic therapy; they are rarely curative and they often complement other therapeutic procedures. A decreased rate of renal excretion is invariably a feature of edematous states. This applies regardless of the underlying pathogenesis of the disease—whether cardiac, hepatic, renal or of some other etiology. Sodium, chloride and bicarbonate are quantitatively the most important ions of the extracellular fluid, and, of these, it is primarily the regulation of sodium excretion that is disturbed in the pathogenesis of edema.

The action of osmotic diuretics (e.g., mannitol) depends upon the increased concentration of osmotically active solutes in the glomerular filtrate. These agents increase the rate of urine flow by reducing the reabsorption of water and, secondarily, of sodium and chloride ions in the proximal tubule. Since the terminal segments of the distal nephron have a compensatory mechanism (mediated by aldosterone) for the decreased reabsorption of sodium in the proximal tubule, a water diuresis without significant sodium loss can occur. Mannitol is effective, so that urine volume can be maintained, even in the presence of decreased glomerular function. It is necessary to administer mannitol solution intravenously, since biological membranes, excluding the glomerular filtration membrane, are relatively impermeable to this compound.

Acetazolamide, a carbonic anhydrase inhibitor, has a diversity of effects in the body, which may be attributed to the widespread distribution of its enzyme receptor site, and there are a variety of therapeutic indications for its use. The diuretic effect of this drug is related to the decrease in supply of hydrogen ions in renal tubule cells for exchange with sodium in the glomerular filtrate. It exerts an important quantitative effect on sodium bicarbonate reabsorption in the proximal tubule. The urine contains more sodium than usual, and there is an elevated potassium ion concentration (potassium is secreted in cortical collecting tubule), together with bicarbonate anion. The increased electrolyte excretion is accompanied by an osmotic equivalent of water. The urine becomes alkaline, and after a short course of therapy metabolic acidosis develops, which is accompanied by loss of the diuretic response. Although they undoubtedly are effective in evoking diuresis, the carbonic anhydrase inhibitors are relatively ineffective compared to agents that act on the ascending limb of Henle's loop. Acetazolamide, which may be given (orally) to reduce intraocular pressure in the management of glaucoma, appears to act at this site independently of systemic acid-base balance (Maren, 1967). It is also considered to be an effective agent for controlling petit mal epilepsy. Acetazolamide is eliminated completely by a combination of renal mechanisms.

The most important locus of action of furosemide and ethacrynic acid is the medullary and diluting segments of the thick ascending limb of Henle's loop, where they inhibit the active reabsorption from tubular fluid of chloride ion—i.e., these diuretic agents block an active electrogenic chloride pump (Burg et al., 1973; Burg and Green, 1973). Inhibition of chloride reabsorption causes a reduction in the uptake (passive) of sodium ion. The medullary thick ascending limb of Henle is completely impermeable to water and urea, relatively impermeable to chloride and moderately permeable to sodium (Kokko, 1974). Inhibition of electrolyte reabsorption has also been observed in the proximal tubule (Morgan et al., 1970). Extracellular fluid volume appears to be the most critical factor in determining the magnitude of the diuretic response. Unlike the organic mercurials and the inhibitors of carbonic anhydrase, the diuretic response to furosemide and ethacrynic acid is largely independent of acid-base balance. The urine contains chloride as the major anion, balanced mostly by sodium and variable amounts of potassium. The increase in potassium excretion results from its secretion in the distal tubule and is approximately proportional to the increased rate of flow in this segment (Duarte et al., 1971). Metabolic alkalosis may be produced and is attributable to the following factors: the loss of chloride and potassium in urine and the increase in rate of hydrogen ion excretion. The diuretic effect of furosemide is additive to that of most diuretic agents, but not ethacrynic acid (Hook and Williamson, 1965). This supports the concept that both furosemide and ethacrynic acid act in a similar manner. One of the major differences between furosemide and ethacrynic acid is that the former has a broader dose–response curve. Accordingly, the therapeutic regimen may be initiated with rather smaller doses and adjusted upward to meet the needs of the individual patient (Mudge, 1975).

It is interesting to compare qualitatively the fate of furosemide and ethacrynic acid. Renal excretion is the principal process of elimination of furosemide (Calesnick et al., 1966). Since the drug is 95 per cent bound to plasma proteins and the renal clearance value in normal human subjects exceeds the rate of glomerular filtration, it may be stated that the renal mechanisms include glomerular filtration and tubular secretion (Cutler et al., 1974). Furosemide excretion by the isolated perfused kidney has been shown to be predominantly a secretory phenomenon (Bowman, 1975). The extensive binding of circulating furosemide to plasma albumin appears to play a significant role in determining the rate at which the drug is secreted. A major advantage of furosemide over organic mercurial and thiazide diuretics is its ability to induce diuresis in patients with advanced renal failure (Allison and Kennedy, 1971; Levin, 1971). Body clearance of furosemide is significantly reduced in functionally anephric patients, owing mainly to a decrease in the overall rate of elimination (half-life is increased). The decreased binding of furosemide to albumin in plasma of uremic patients (Andreasen and Jakobsen, 1974) increases the amount of drug available in the plasma for distribution and excretion by passive processes. Nonrenal elimination mechanisms are unimpaired in uremic patients without liver disease and become the principal means of furosemide clearance in patients with advanced renal failure (Huang et al., 1974). Ethacrynic acid is eliminated by a combination of processes of biotransformation and excretion, both renal and biliary. Beyer and co-workers (1965) reported that 35 per cent or less of the drug was excreted in the urine of rats and dogs, regardless of mode of administration, and that 50 per cent or more appeared in feces, suggesting hepatic elimination of the drug. About 20 to 30 per cent of the drug excreted into the urine appeared to be a cysteine adduct of ethacrynic acid. A portion (about 20 per cent in rats and 40 per cent in dogs) of the drug in bile is in the unchanged form, and the remainder is biotransformation products (Klaassen and Fitzgerald, 1974). The major metabolites in bile were the glutathione and cysteine (dog only) adducts and ethacrynic acid–mercapturate. The unchanged ethacrynic acid excreted into bile and that derived from the reconversion of metabolites (conjugates) by intestinal flora probably undergo enterohepatic circulation, since ethacrynic acid is well absorbed from the intestine. Unfortunately inadequate data are available at the present time to make a quantitative comparison of the fate of furosemide and ethacrynic acid in any single species.

The distal nephron is composed of several tubule segments in series which differ in their microscopic anatomy and ion transport mechanisms (Burg and Stoner, 1974). The first segment, called the "diluting segment," begins at the point in the thick ascending limb of the loop of Henle where it crosses from the outer medulla into the cortex. In mammals the diluting segment extends to the macula densa. The distal convoluted tubule extends from the macula densa to the peripheral junctions where it joins other distal tubules to form the cortical collecting tubules. The fourth segment is the papillary collecting duct. In each segment there is net sodium chloride reabsorption. Active chloride reabsorption predominates in the diluting segment. Sodium transport in this segment is largely or entirely passive. Active sodium transport predominates in the other segments, although there is also active potassium (and possibly chloride) reabsorption in the distal convoluted tubule, and active potassium secretion in the cortical collecting tubule. Control of the dilution and concentration of the urine and the excretion of potassium occurs in the distal nephron. This region of the nephron is the site of action of hormones such as antidiuretic hormone (ADH) and aldosterone, and of various diuretic agents. Water permeability is low in the diluting segment and is variable in the other segments, depending on the presence of ADH. This hormone causes the water permeability of the distal convoluted tubule and terminal segments to increase greatly.

The high-ceiling diuretics, namely, furosemide and ethacrynic acid, inhibit active chloride transport in the diluting segment and thus decrease markedly the reabsorption of sodium chloride. The thiazides act in the distal convoluted tubule where they inhibit the active reabsorption of sodium and, consequently, increase the renal excretion of sodium chloride with an accompanying volume of water. Like furosemide and ethacrynic acid but unlike the mercurials and carbonic anhydrase inhibitors, the action of thiazides is virtually independent of acid-base balance. The thiazides evoke a significant augmentation of potassium excretion in amounts sufficient to produce hypokalemia. The decreased sodium reabsorption stimulates the sodium-potassium exchange mechanism of the terminal segments, which is mediated by aldosterone, in an attempt to conserve sodium at the expense of potassium, which is secreted. The thiazides vary widely in their potency as inhibitors of carbonic anhydrase and cause variable losses of bicarbonate in urine. The thiazides tend, however, to produce less distortion in the extracellular fluid composition than do other diuretic agents. It should be emphasized that all thiazides so far extensively examined have parallel dose–response curves and comparable maximal chloruretic effects. This implies that they have a similar mechanism of action. The various analogues differ primarily in the dose required to produce a given effect (i.e., potency) and do not necessarily differ with respect to their optimal therapeutic response. The thiazides are excreted unchanged in urine by a combination of renal mechanisms. Thiazides should be a part of all antihypertensive dosage regimens. The combination of reserpine (or its equivalent, rauwolfia) and a thiazide is effective in almost all patients with mild hypertension and in most patients with moderate hypertension (Smith et al., 1964, 1969). Methyldopa is especially valuable in hypertensive patients with compromised renal function. Guanethidine is most useful in moderate-to-severe hypertension, but may be given in small doses to patients with mild hypertension which is not controlled by other drugs, or to those who cannot tolerate other drugs.

Potassium-sustaining agents appear to inhibit the sodium-potassium exchange mechanism in the distal nephron (cortical collecting tubules) either by competitively antagonizing the tubular action of aldosterone (e.g., spironolactone) or by interfering directly with tubular transport (e.g., triamterene, amiloride). Spironolactone is a true competitive antagonist of aldosterone. It depresses the sodium-potassium exchange mechanism mainly by reducing the secretion of K^+, but also through the reabsorption of sodium. Spironolactone has limited diuretic activity when compared with agents that act on the diluting segment and distal convoluted tubule (thiazides). Triamterene reduces the rate of potassium secretion in the distal nephron, presumably the cortical collecting tubules, somewhat indirectly. The effect is achieved by a primary reduction in sodium reabsorption, which in turn leads to a drop in the transtubular electrical potential difference. It is the latter that is normally the driving force for potassium secretion (Gatzy, 1971). Triamterene is uniquely valuable in the treatment of "pseudoaldosteronism" (a familial renal disorder characterized by hypertension, hypokalemia and subnormal aldosterone secretion) by virtue of the fact that, unlike spironolactone, it promotes sodium excretion and potassium conservation in the absence of aldosterone as well as in its presence (Liddle, 1966).

The use of spironolactone or triamterene in conjunction with a thiazide represents one of the few rational drug combinations, but the electrolyte status must be monitored. Spironolactone and triamterene are available in oral dosage forms only. In the treatment of congestive heart failure, digitalization and this form of diuretic therapy is a reasonable approach.

Influence of Renal Disease on Drug Disposition

Renal disease can influence the distribution and elimination of drugs in various ways, so that the intensity and duration of pharmacological activity can be altered while potential toxicity is invariably increased. The binding of many drugs to albumin is decreased in plasma of uremic patients. In patients with chronic renal disease, the rates of some metabolic reactions are decreased, the overall elimination rate of all drugs excreted unchanged to a substantial degree by the kidneys is reduced (their half-lives are markedly increased), and tissue (CNS) sensitivity to some drugs (e.g., barbiturates, narcotics) is increased. Any of these alterations in drug disposition that occur in uremia may lead to adverse drug reactions unless the usual dosage regimen is modified. Immunologic responsiveness in chronic renal disease is abnormal (Lawrence, 1965; Wilson et al., 1965). Lymphocyte function and survival in chronic renal failure have been demonstrated to be impaired.

The extent of drug binding to plasma albumin may be decreased in patients with renal disease. Many of the drugs which show reduced binding are organic acids (Table 5–4). For drugs that are extensively bound to plasma proteins, decrease in the extent of their binding may

Table 5-4 DRUGS WHICH SHOW DECREASED BINDING TO
ALBUMIN IN PLASMA OF UREMIC PATIENTS

Drug	Reference
Phenytoin (diphenylhydantoin)	Reidenberg et al. (1971); Baggot and Davis (1973 a); Hooper et al. (1974)
Pentobarbital	Ehrnebo and Odar-Cederlöf (1975)
Phenylbutazone	Andreasen (1973); Mussche et al. (1975)
Sulfamethazine	Anton and Corey (1971)
Diazoxide	O'Malley et al. (1975)
Furosemide	Andreasen and Jakobsen (1974)
Cardiac glycosides	Baggot and Davis (1973 b)

cause profound alterations in their disposition and pharmacodynamic
behavior. The increase in fraction of the drug in plasma that is free
means that more drug is available for distribution and excretion
processes, which are of a passive nature, so that a lower fraction of
the dose is present in the plasma, the volume of distribution is
increased, and a greater pharmacological response may be obtained.
Most of the present analytical techniques measure the total (free +
bound) drug concentration in the plasma. Therapeutic plasma levels
of drugs quoted in the literature usually refer to the total drug concentration, while pharmacological activity is associated only with the
fraction of the drug in plasma that is free—i.e., dissolved in plasma
water. Consequently, the usual dose of a drug may give lower (total)
plasma levels but indicate increased pharmacological activity, which
could be interpreted as increased tissue sensitivity, in patients with
acute or chronic renal failure or nephrosis. The basic drugs—morphine, amphetamine, quinidine and desmethylimipramine—bind normally in plasma from uremic subjects, while triamterene binding is
decreased (Reidenberg and Affrime, 1973). For drugs whose binding
is decreased in uremia, there is no consistent correlation between the
extent of binding reduction and the severity of renal insufficiency, as
reflected by serum creatinine or blood urea nitrogen concentrations
(Hooper et al., 1974; Olsen et al., 1975; O'Malley et al., 1975). The
increase of the free drug fraction in the plasma of patients with renal
disease does correlate with the degree of hypoalbuminemia, but is not
fully explained by it (Reidenberg et al., 1971; Andreasen, 1973;
Hooper et al., 1974; Olsen et al., 1975; O'Malley et al., 1975). Other
factors which could contribute to the decreased interaction of drugs
and albumin in renal failure include conformational changes in the albumin molecule that decrease its drug-binding capacity or the accumulation in the plasma of drug metabolites or endogenous substances that compete with drugs for binding sites on albumin

(Dromgoole, 1974; Andreasen, 1974; Andreasen and Jakobsen, 1974).

The metabolism of drugs by certain pathways is slowed in uremia (Reidenberg, 1971). These pathways include acetylation of sulfisoxazole (Reidenberg et al., 1969), the reduction of cortisol (Englert et al., 1958) and the hydrolysis of esters such as procaine, metabolized by plasma pseudocholinesterase (Reidenberg et al., 1972). The available evidence suggests that the concentration of plasma pseudocholinesterase is low in uremia, not that the enzyme is inhibited by some unexcreted waste product. The usual dosage regimens of drugs with narrow therapeutic indices that are eliminated predominantly by metabolic pathways that are impaired in uremia would have to be modified for patients with renal disease to avoid excessive cumulation and toxicity. Drug oxidation reactions and glucuronide conjugation, metabolic pathways that are mediated by the hepatic microsomal enzyme systems, appear to be normal in uremia (Reidenberg, 1971). In humans, lidocaine is metabolized by hydrolysis and N-dealkylation (Keenaghan and Boyes, 1972). Plasma lidocaine levels above 1.4 μg/ml generally are effective in reducing the frequency of premature ventricular contractions and suppressing ventricular tachycardia; toxic reactions increase as plasma levels exceed 6.0 μg/ml (Gianelly et al., 1967; Harrison et al., 1970). It is important that the plasma lidocaine concentration be maintained within this range of levels. Fortunately, lidocaine pharmacokinetics in uremic patients are similar to those in normal subjects (Collinsworth et al., 1975). Depressed renal function does not alter the overall rate of elimination of pentobarbital (Davis et al., 1973). This drug is eliminated entirely by hepatic biotransformation (oxidation and conjugation). However, uremia may increase the sensitivity of a patient to the hypnotic effects of barbiturates (Richards et al., 1953) due, at least in part, to a decreased extent of binding of these organic acids to plasma albumin. The plasma half-life of antipyrine is widely used as an index of drug oxidation. The mean ($\pm$ S.D.) plasma antipyrine half-life in patients with chronic renal failure (7.3$\pm$2.0 hours) was significantly shorter than in normal subjects (13.2 $\pm$4.3 hours; p $<$ 0.002). There was no statistical difference in the apparent volume of distribution of the drug between the two groups (Maddocks et al., 1975). The diminished plasma antipyrine half-life in patients with chronic renal failure is attributed to increased oxidative metabolism of the drug by hepatic microsomal enzymes.

Examination of the changes in disposition of phenytoin that occur in various conditions is instructive. Phenytoin is extensively ($>$ 75 per cent) bound to plasma proteins, mainly albumin. The percentage of total drug in the plasma that is free increases with phenytoin concentration, even within the therapeutic range (10 to 20 μg/ml). A greater fraction is free in neonates, in patients with hypoalbuminemia and in uremic patients (Rane et al., 1971; Reidenberg et al., 1971; Hooper et al., 1974). Biotransformation is the principal process of elimination, and over 95 per cent of the dose is metabolized by the hepatic microsomal enzyme systems. The rate of elimination of phenytoin is dose-dependent, perhaps because the hydroxylation reaction approaches saturation or is inhibited by the metabolites. At plasma concentrations below 10 μg/ml, elimination is exponential (first-order); there is, however, wide individual variation in half-life. A small dose (2 mg/kg) of phenytoin was infused intravenously in four uremic patients and four healthy volunteers and its plasma concentration (total phenytoin) measured during and after the infusion (Odar-Cederlöf and Borga, 1974). The plasma concentrations were considerably lower in the uremic subjects, and the apparent volume of distribution was higher. These observations could be explained by the lower plasma protein binding of phenytoin in the uremic patients. The overall elimination rate constant was larger (shorter half-life) in the presence of uremia. The increased rate of elimination could not be explained by reduced plasma protein binding, but it might be due to induction of phenytoin metabolism in the uremic state.

The most profound consequence of renal disease on drug disposition and action is the decrease in rate of elimination of polar drugs and drug metabolites which have pharmacological activity. This is reflected by an increase in the half-life values of these drugs and excessive accumulation, giving rise to signs of toxicity, when dosed according to the usual regimens. The margin of safety (therapeutic index) and dosage regimen applied determine the potential toxicity of each individual compound. Most antibiotics, with the exceptions of chloramphenicol, doxycycline, erythromycin and clindamycin, are eliminated almost entirely unchanged by renal excretion. Glomerular filtration is the renal mechanism for excretion of these drugs, except for penicillins, which also undergo carrier-mediated tubular excretion (secretion). The sulfonamides, trimethoprim and nitrofurantoin are eliminated by a combination of biotransformation and renal excretion processes. The renal handling of sulfonamides and contribution of renal excretion to overall elimination depend on the pK_a, degree of lipid solubility and extent of binding to plasma albumin of the individual sulfonamide compound. The effectiveness of antimicrobial therapy depends largely on the susceptibility of the invading microorganisms to the unchanged drug level attained at the source of infection. Since nitrofurantoin is eliminated both by renal excretion (glomerular filtration) and by biotransformation, an ineffective level of the drug will be present in the urine of patients with delayed excretion (Sachs et al., 1968). Moreover, the elevated plasma levels in uremic patients may cause neurotoxicity. Doxycycline is a safe and effective compound for use when a tetracycline is indicated for the therapy of systemic infection complicating preexisting renal disease (Whelton et al., 1974). Although the state of hydration, the urine pH and renal disease all influence significantly the urinary concentrations and rate of excretion of doxycycline, the same concentrations of the antibiotic are attained in severely diseased kidneys as in normal renal tissue (Whelton et al., 1975). This result is in contradistinction to the finding for penicillins (Whelton et al., 1971, 1972, 1973), cephalosporins (Whelton et al., 1971) and aminoglycosides (Whelton and Walker, 1974). When drug concentrations in normal kidneys were compared with those achievable through similar dosage schedules in severely diseased human kidneys, a marked reduction in the renal accumulation of penicillins, cephalosporins and aminoglycosides was noted. At therapeutic levels in serum, drugs other than doxycycline exhibit levels in diseased renal parenchymal tissue that range from 0.85 to 0.5 of the concomitant serum level of the drug in question. The level of doxycycline in renal tissue averages twice the concentration in serum without notable difference among levels in renal cortex, medulla and papilla (Whelton et al., 1975). The therapeutic significance of doxycycline accumulation in diseased renal parenchymal tissue remains to be evaluated.

The use of diuretics is not recommended in patients with renal disease (Kessler, 1965; Hunt and Maher, 1966). Since diuretic agents interfere with tubular reabsorption of electrolytes, their effectiveness decreases as renal function deteriorates (Reubi and Coltier, 1961). Furosemide is the most effective and least toxic diuretic in patients with advanced renal failure. Larger doses are required to induce diuresis, since the diuretic response is adversely affected by poor renal function and dehydration (Muth, 1971; Allison and Kennedy, 1971). For maximal efficacy in uremic patients, furosemide should be given by slow intravenous infusion (Huang et al., 1974). Renal excretion is the principal process of furosemide elimination in subjects with normal renal function. The half-life of the drug is markedly prolonged in patients with advanced renal failure. Renal furosemide clearance is reduced, but elimination by nonrenal mechanisms is unimpaired in uremic patients without liver disease (Cutler et al., 1974). The major site of nonrenal elimination is probably the liver. The renal clearance of furosemide in dogs decreases proportionately with progressive azotemia and is not related to the renal blood flow or exogenous urea or metabolite (Rose et al., 1976). The degree of azotemia was measured as the blood urea nitrogen (BUN) concentration, although an elevated

BUN is not the most significant physiological abnormality of azotemia (Preuss et al., 1966). However, if actual BUN concentration is plotted against clearance of furosemide, it appears that there is a linear relationship between the BUN level in the serum and its ability to depress furosemide transport. The renal tubular secretion of furosemide shares the classical characteristics of the organic acid system. The defective tubular secretion of furosemide in azotemia, due probably to competitive inhibition by accumulated organic acids in plasma of uremic patients, may account in part for the reduced therapeutic efficacy of the diuretic agent in renal disease accompanied by azotemia.

When treating patients with renal disease, it is essential to give special consideration to dosages of drugs that have a relatively narrow margin of safety and are eliminated substantially unchanged by renal mechanisms in normal subjects. Therapeutic substances which fall into this category include cardiac glycosides, procainamide and aminoglycoside antibiotics (gentamicin, kanamycin, streptomycin). The use of guanethidine probably should be avoided in hypertensive patients with renal disease.

Biliary Excretion

Blood from the portal vein and hepatic artery flows into liver sinusoids, lined by reticuloendothelial cells, that lie between cords of hepatocytes (liver parenchymal cells). It is by means of the sinusoids that blood circulates through the liver, enabling the hepatocytes of the cords to have a means of obtaining nutrients and of disposing waste products (including drug metabolites), as well as secreting certain of their products (e.g., glucose, plasma albumin) into the bloodstream. Bile is an exocrine secretion of hepatocytes. The bile is secreted into canaliculi and flows along between the hepatocytes of a cord of cells, finally entering a bile duct in a portal tract. Bile contains pigments (bilirubin), bile salts, protein, cholesterol and such crystalloids (dissolved in water) as are present in tissue fluid. Bilirubin pigment is primarily a waste product. It is formed not in hepatic cells, but from breakdown of the hemoglobin of erythrocytes by the macrophages that are closely associated with the sinusoids of the spleen and the bone marrow and, to a lesser extent, by the Kupffer cells of hepatic sinusoids. The circulating bilirubin passes into hepatocytes, where it is conjugated and thereby made water-soluble. The conjugate bilirubin glucuronide is secreted by the hepatocytes into bile. Steroid hormones produced by the adrenal cortex and sex glands are constantly absorbed from the blood by hepatocytes and metabolized to different extents. The metabolic products, and even active unchanged steroid

Table 5–5   THE pH REACTION AND RATE OF SECRETION OF BILE*

Species	pH of Gallbladder Bile	Rate of Secretion (ml/kg/day)
Horse	Absent	21
Ox	6.7 –7.5	15
Sheep	6.0 –6.7	12
Dog	5.18–6.97	12
Cat	5.0 –6.0	14

*Data from Altman and Dittmer (1961): *Blood and Other Body Fluids.* Washington, D.C., Federation of American Societies for Experimental Biology.

hormones, are partly secreted into bile. Current concepts indicate that bile flow is the result of secretory activity of the hepatic parenchymal cells lining the bile canaliculi. The pH reaction of gallbladder bile and daily rate of secretion in various species of domestic animals are tabulated in Table 5–5.

Although the principal route of excretion of most drugs and their metabolites is through the kidney into the urine, some compounds are excreted partly or mainly through the liver into bile. The biliary excretion of a compound may take place by passive diffusion of drug molecules from hepatic sinusoids through the parenchymal cells into bile. A large number of drugs are excreted to a small extent (about 5 per cent of the dose) by this mechanism. The hepatic sinusoids are bounded by reticuloendothelium, which consists of a porous endothelial membrane with interspersed Kupffer cells. Most unbound circulating drug molecules, whether in the hepatic portal vein or systemic circulation, can enter the hepatocytes, which are the principal site of biotransformation of lipid-soluble compounds. The molecular weight and polarity of the compounds will determine whether they diffuse passively into blood and bile or are transported actively into bile. The active transfer systems require the expenditure of energy and are carrier-mediated. It appears that polar compounds, which may be drugs, drug metabolites (in particular glucuronide conjugates) and endogenous substances, with molecular weights in excess of 300 are likely to be excreted in bile in significant amounts (Table 5–6). Clearance of Bromsulphalein (BSP) is widely used to assess hepatic function in domestic animals (Cornelius, 1970). The major portion of BSP is conjugated in the liver with glutathione and excreted in bile (Grodsky et al., 1959).

Generally, with compounds of molecular weight less than 300, there is little variation in the extent of their biliary excretion among species, even though there could be a species variation in the nature of the biliary metabolites (Abou-El-Makarem et al., 1967). When the

Table 5–6 COMPOUNDS THAT UNDERGO BILIARY EXCRETION

Unchanged Drugs and Endogenous Substances	Compounds Excreted as Glucuronide Conjugates
Erythromycin	Chloramphenicol
Clindamycin	Trimethoprim
Digitoxin	Sulfadimethoxine (N^1—)
Iopanoic acid	Glutethimide
Bromsulphalein	Morphine
Steroid hormones	Bilirubin
Bile acids	Thyroxine
	Stilbestrol

molecular weight of a polar compound is between 300 and 500, species variation in the extent of biliary excretion is likely to occur. Species may be classified as "good" (rats, dogs, chickens), "moderate" (cats, sheep) or "poor" (guinea pigs, rabbits, Rhesus monkeys and probably humans) biliary excretors (Williams, 1971). This classification of species is based on the minimum molecular weight for the extensive biliary excretion of polar compounds. The slow rate of synthesis of glucuronide conjugates in cats must contribute to the lower extent of biliary excretion of many compounds in this species compared with that in dogs. Excretion in the bile is an important route for elimination of organic anions and cations of molecular weight above 500 (e.g., Bromsulphalein, iopanoic acid) in all species.

Compounds excreted in bile are conveyed ultimately into the small intestine. Polar drugs will, for the most part, be excreted in the feces. Glucuronide conjugates, both of drugs (e.g., morphine, chloramphenicol) and of endogenous substances (e.g., stilbestrol, bilirubin), may be hydrolyzed by enzymes in the gastrointestinal microflora to liberate the parent lipid-soluble compound or a somewhat less lipid-soluble phase I metabolite. The liberated compound may be reabsorbed, excreted or reduced prior to excretion in the feces. When the physicochemical properties of the compound in the intestine are favorable for absorption by passive diffusion, an enterohepatic cycle will be established (Fig. 5–3). This term implies the excretion of a compound by hepatocytes into bile, passage into the small intestine, absorption into portal venous blood and return to hepatic sinusoids. The pharmacological significance of an enterohepatic circulation for a drug depends on the fraction of the dose excreted in bile. When the amount is substantial, the effects of a single dose of the drug will be prolonged (e.g., digitoxin) and reflected in the overall elimination rate constant. The main importance of biliary excretion as a mechanism of drug elimination is in clearance of organic anions and cations that are

ENTEROHEPATIC CIRCULATION OF A DRUG

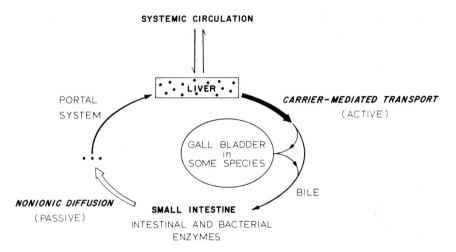

Figure 5–3   The enterohepatic circulation of a lipid-soluble foreign or endogenous compound. Glucuronide conjugates, excreted in bile, may be hydrolyzed in the
small intestine and the liberated parent compound may be reabsorbed.

highly ionized and have low lipid-solubility. A drug with this combination of physicochemical properties can only be poorly absorbed
from the small intestine, as drug absorption is a passive diffusion
process.

Salivary Excretion

Whereas biliary excretion is the main process by which polar
drugs and metabolites, which may be reactivated, are transported into
the gastrointestinal tract, salivary excretion and passive diffusion
across the gastrointestinal (and reticuloruminal) mucosa are avenues
for excretion of weak organic electrolytes. Transport of organic acids
and bases from blood plasma into saliva is similar to passage of drugs
into milk and takes place by the process of nonionic diffusion. The
most important factors that govern penetration of organic electrolytes
into saliva are the degree of lipid-solubility of the drug, the concentration of the nonionized moiety that is free in the plasma, and the
salivary pH reaction. Ruminants secrete considerably larger volumes
of saliva than animals with simple stomachs, and ruminant saliva has

a significantly higher pH and bicarbonate ion concentration. Ruminant saliva is alkaline (pH 8.0 to 8.4), saliva of horses (pH 7.3 to 7.6), dogs and cats is nearly neutral and human saliva is somewhat acidic (pH 6.5 to 7.2). Variations in the rate of secretion and pH of saliva among species cause quantitative differences in salivary excretion of weak organic electrolytes. In the alkaline saliva of cows and goats, weak acids such as sulfadiazine (pK_a 6.5), sulfamethazine (pK_a 7.4), phenobarbitone (pK_a 7.2) and pentobarbitone (pK_a 8.0) were present in concentrations higher than their unbound levels in plasma (Rasmussen, 1964). Sulfacetamide (pK 5.4), which is predominantly ionized (99 per cent) in blood plasma and has a low degree of lipid-solubility, did not attain its predicted saliva-to-plasma concentration ratio. By comparison, the slightly acid saliva of humans contained sulfonamides and barbiturates in concentrations lower than the unbound fractions of these drugs in the plasma (Killmann and Thaysen, 1955). Alexander and Nicholson (1968) showed that in horses the concentrations of phenobarbitone and pentobarbitone in the saliva were directly dependent on the non-plasma protein–bound barbiturate concentrations. The apparent conflict between this conclusion and the hypothesis of other investigators (Thaysen and Schwartz, 1953; Killmann and Thaysen, 1955; Rasmussen, 1964), who have found that it is the nonionized drug concentration in the plasma that governs the salivary concentration, is readily explained by the equality in pH between horse plasma and saliva (Alexander, 1966). The saliva-to-plasma ratio for digoxin concentration in humans is 0.78 (Huffman, 1975). Since digoxin binding to plasma proteins is 23 per cent (Lukas and DeMartino, 1969), it is apparent that it is the free digoxin in the plasma that is in equilibrium with the saliva. Antipyrine (a base with pK_a of 1.4) is an analgesic-antipyretic that distributes evenly in total body water (Soberman et al., 1949), does not bind to plasma proteins, is excreted in urine entirely as conjugated metabolite (Brodie and Axelrod, 1950) and appears in measurable quantities in saliva (DeAngelis and Welch, 1974). Since the elimination of antipyrine is totally dependent on its metabolism by the liver, the plasma half-life of antipyrine is a useful index of hepatic metabolism of drugs in animals and humans. Since the distribution ratio of antipyrine between saliva and plasma is essentially 1 in rats and humans following administration of an oral or parenteral dose of the drug, the elimination rate (biological half-life) of antipyrine may be determined by measuring the salivary concentration of the drug (Welch et al., 1975). In goats, trimethoprim undergoes extensive hepatic biotransformation, but excretion processes (renal, biliary and to a lesser extent salivary) also contribute to its rapid removal from the body. More than 99 per cent of the amount excreted in bile consists of metabolites of trimethoprim. In contrast, it is almost exclusively the unchanged drug that is excreted in the saliva (Nielsen and Rasmussen, 1976). The concentrations of trimethoprim and metabolites in ruminal fluid were much lower than in the plasma, while the concentrations in abomasum were two to five times higher than in the plasma. The relative amounts of metabolites in both rumen and abomasum were much lower than those found in the urine and bile. Passive diffusion of lipid-soluble organic bases into ruminal fluid is a feature of their distribution in cattle, sheep and goats, so that apparent specific volumes of distribution of these drugs may be substantially higher in ruminant animals than in monogastric species. Passage of lipophilic drugs from the systemic circulation into gastrointestinal fluids is not restricted to ruminant species. Doxycycline is a long-acting tetracycline antibiotic, which, in humans at least, is eliminated from the systemic circulation by passive diffusion into the luminal contents of the small intestine (Whelton et al., 1974). In the lumen, cationic chelation occurs and in such form doxycycline cannot be reabsorbed and is excreted in the feces. Minor additional contributions to fecal elimination of the drug are made by biliary excretion. As a result of the mechanisms for elimination of doxycycline, this antibiotic may be administered at usual dosage regimen when a tetracycline is indicated for the therapy of systemic infections in anephric patients or in the presence of renal impairment, since the extension of the drug's biological (or plasma) half-life is not clinically significant.

A drug that is excreted in saliva or diffuses directly into gastrointestinal fluids may be reabsorbed by passive diffusion, be chemically inactivated by gastric acidity, be metabolized by ruminal or intestinal microorganisms or be excreted unchanged in the feces. Absorption is the most likely fate of drugs that enter the gastrointestinal tract via the saliva. During the process of absorption, enzymes located in the intestinal mucosa may inactivate a fraction of the drug molecules. The fraction absorbed must pass through the liver before reentering the systemic circulation.

REFERENCES

Abou-El-Makarem, M. M., Millburn, P., Smith, R. L., and Williams, R. T. (1967): Biliary excretion of foreign compounds. *Biochem. J., 105*:1289–1293.

Alexander, F. (1966): A study of parotid salivation in the horse. *J. Physiol.* (Lond.), *184*:646–656.

Alexander, F., and Nicholson, J. D. (1968): The blood and saliva clearances of phenobarbitone and pentobarbitone in the horse. *Biochem. Pharmacol., 17*:203–210.

Allison, M. E., and Kennedy, A. C. (1971): Diuretics in chronic renal disease: A study of high dosage furosemide. *Clin. Sci., 41*:171–187.

Altman, P. L., and Dittmer, D. S. (1961): *Blood and Other Body Fluids.* Washington, D.C., Federation of American Societies for Experimental Biology.

Andreasen, F. (1973): Protein binding of drugs in plasma from patients with acute renal failure. *Acta Pharmacol. Toxicol., 32*:417–429.

Andreasen, F. (1974): The effect of dialysis on the protein binding of drugs in the plasma of patients with acute renal failure. *Acta Pharmacol. Toxicol., 34*:284–294.

Andreasen, F., and Jakobsen, P. (1974): Determination of furosemide in blood plasma and its binding to proteins in normal plasma and in plasma from patients with acute renal failure. *Acta Pharmacol. Toxicol., 35*:49–57.

Anton, A. H., and Corey, W. T. (1971): Interindividual differences in the protein binding of sulfonamides: The effect of disease and drugs. *Acta Pharmacol. Toxicol., 29* (Suppl. 3): 134–151.

Asheim, A., Persson, F., and Persson, S. (1961): Renal clearance in dogs with regard to variations according to age and sex. *Acta physiol. scand., 51*:150–162.

Baggot, J. D., and Davis, L. E. (1973a): Comparative study of plasma protein binding of diphenylhydantoin. *Comp. gen. Pharmacol., 4*:399–404.

Baggot, J. D., and Davis, L. E. (1973b): Plasma protein binding of digitoxin and digoxin in several mammalian species. *Res. vet. Sci., 15*:81–87.

Beyer, K. H., Baer, J. E., Michaelson, J. K., and Russo, H. F. (1965): Renotropic characteristics of ethacrynic acid: A phenoxyacetic saluretic-diuretic agent. *J. Pharmacol. exp. Ther., 147*:1–22.

Bowman, R. H. (1975): Renal secretion of [^{35}S] furosemide and its depression by albumin binding. *Am. J. Physiol., 229*:93–98.

Brodie, B. B., and Axelrod, J. (1950): The fate of antipyrine in man. *J. Pharmacol. Exp. Ther., 98*:97–104.

Burg, M. B., and Green, N. (1973): Effect of ethacrynic acid on the thick ascending limb of Henle's loop. *Kidney Internat., 4*:301–308.

Burg, M., and Stoner, L. (1974): Sodium transport in the distal nephron. *Fed. Proc., 33*:31–36.

Burg, M. B., Stoner, L., Cardinal, J., and Green, N. (1973): Furosemide effect on isolated perfused tubules. *Am. J. Physiol., 225*:119–124.

Calesnick, B., Christensen, L. J., and Richter, N. (1966): Absorption and excretion of furosemide S^{35} in human subjects. *Proc. Soc. exp. Biol. Med., 123*:17–22.

Chiou, W. L., and Hsu, F. H. (1975): Pharmacokinetics of creatinine in man and its implications in the monitoring of renal function and in dosage regimen modifications in patients with renal insufficiency. *J. clin. Pharmacol., 15*:427–434.

Collinsworth, K. A., Strong, J. M., Atkinson, A. J., Winkle, R. A., Perlroth, F., and Harrison, D. C. (1975): Pharmacokinetics and metabolism of lidocaine in patients with renal failure. *Clin. Pharmacol. Ther., 18*:59–64.

Cornelius, C. E. (1970): Liver function. *In* J. J. Kaneko and C. E. Cornelius (eds.): *Clinical Biochemistry of Domestic Animals.* Vol. 1, 2nd Ed. New York, Academic Press, pp. 161–230.

Cutler, R. E., Forrey, A. W., Christopher, T. G., and Kimpel, B. M. (1974): Pharmacokinetics of furosemide in normal subjects and functionally anephric patients. *Clin. Pharmacol. Ther., 15*:588–596.

Davis, L. E., Baggot, J. D., Neff-Davis, C. A., and Powers, T. E. (1973): Elimination kinetics of pentobarbital in nephrectomized dogs. *Am. J. vet. Res., 34*:231–233.

DeAngelis, R. L., and Welch, R. M. (1974): The salivary half-life of antipyrine as a convenient measure of drug metabolism in man [abstr.]. *Fed. Proc., 33*:534.

Dromgoole, S. H. (1974): The binding capacity of albumin and renal disease. *J. Pharmacol. exp. Ther., 191*:318–323.

Duarte, C. C., Chomety, F., and Giebisch, G. (1971): Effect of amiloride, ouabain, and furosemide on distal tubular function in the rat. *Am. J. Physiol., 221*:632–640.

Ehrnebo, M., and Odar-Cederlöf, I. (1975): Binding of amobarbital, pentobarbital and diphenylhydantoin to blood cells and plasma proteins in healthy volunteers and uraemic patients. *Europ. J. clin. Pharmacol., 8*:445–453.

Englert, E., Brown, H., Willardson, D. G., Wallach, S., and Simons, E. L. (1958): Metabolism of free and conjugated 17-hydroxycorticosteroids in subjects with uremia. *J. clin. Endocr., 18*:36–48.

Finco, D. R., and Duncan, J. R. (1976): Evaluation of blood urea nitrogen and serum creatinine concentrations as indicators of renal dysfunction: a study of 111 cases and a review of related literature. *J. Am. vet. med. Ass., 168*:593–601.

Gatzy, J. T. (1971): The effect of K⁺-sparing diuretics on ion transport across the excised toad bladder. *J. Pharmacol. exp. Ther., 176*:580–594.

Gianelly, R. E., Von Der Groeben, J. O., Spivack, A. P., and Harrison, D. C. (1967): Effect of lidocaine on ventricular arrhythmias in patients with coronary heart disease. *N. Engl. J. Med., 277*:1215–1219.

Grodsky, G. M., Carbone, J. V., and Fanska, R. (1959): Identification of metabolites of sulfobromophthalein. *J. clin. Invest., 38*:1981–1988.

Gyrd-Hansen, N. (1968): Renal clearances in pigs: inulin, endogenous creatinine, urea, para-aminohippuric acid, sodium, potassium, and chloride. *Acta vet. scand., 9*:183–198.

Harrison, D. C., Stenson, R. E., and Constantino, R. T. (1970): The relationship of blood levels, infusion rates and metabolism of lidocaine to its antiarrhythmic action. *In* E. Sandøe, E. Flensted-Jensen and K. H. Olesen (eds.): *Symposium on Cardiac Arrhythmias.* Södertälje, Sweden, A. B. Astra, pp. 427–447.

Hook, J. B., and Williamson, H. E. (1965): Addition of the saluretic action of furosemide to the saluretic action of certain other agents. *J. Pharmacol. exp. Ther., 148*:88–93.

Hooper, W. D., Bochner, F., Eadie, M. J., and Tyrer, J. H. (1974): Plasma protein binding of diphenylhydantoin: Effects of sex hormones, renal and hepatic disease. *Clin. Pharmacol. Ther., 15*:276–282.

Huang, C. M., Atkinson, A. J., Levin, M., Levin, N. W., and Quintanilla, A. (1974): Pharmacokinetics of furosemide in advanced renal failure. *Clin. Pharmacol. Ther., 16*:659–666.

Huffman, D. H. (1975): Relationship between digoxin concentrations in serum and saliva. *Clin. Pharmacol. Ther., 17*:310–312.

Hunt, J. C., and Maher, F. T. (1966): Diuretic drugs in patients with impaired renal function. *Am. J. Cardiol., 17*:642–647.

Kampmann, J., Molholm Hansen, J., Siersboek-Nielsen, K., and Laursen, H. (1972): Effect of some drugs on penicillin half-life in blood. *Clin. Pharmacol. Ther., 13*:516–519.

Keenaghan, J. B., and Boyes, R. N. (1972): The tissue distribution, metabolism and excretion of lidocaine in rats, guinea pigs, dogs and man. *J. Pharmacol. exp. Ther., 180*:454–463.

Kessler, R. H. (1965): On the use of natriuretic drugs in the treatment of edema due to renal disease. *Clin. Pharmacol. Ther., 6*:1–4.

Killmann, S. A., and Thaysen, J. H. (1955): The permeability of the human parotid gland to a series of sulfonamide compounds, para-aminohippurate and inulin. *Scand. J. clin. lab. Invest., 7*:86–91.

Klaassen, C. D., and Fitzgerald, T. J. (1974): Metabolism and biliary excretion of ethacrynic acid. *J. Pharmacol. exp. Ther., 191*:548–556.

Knudsen, E. (1959): Renal clearance studies on the horse. I. Inulin, endogenous creatinine and urea. *Acta vet scand., 1*:52–66.

Kokko, J. P. (1974): Membrane characteristics governing salt and water transport in the loop of Henle. *Fed. Proc., 33*:25–30.

Lawrence, H. S. (1965): Uremia—nature's immunosuppressive device. *Ann. intern. Med., 62*:166–169.

Levin, N. W. (1971): Furosemide and ethacrynic acid in renal insufficiency. *Med. Clin. N. Amer., 55*:107–120.

Liddle, G. W. (1966): Aldosterone antagonists and triamterene. *Ann. N. Y. Acad. Sci., 139*:466–470.

Lukas, D. S., and DeMartino, A. G. (1969): Binding of digitoxin and some related cardenolides to human plasma proteins. *J. clin. Invest., 48*:1041–1053.

Maddocks, J. L., Wake, C. J., and Harber, M. J. (1975): The plasma half-life of antipyrine in chronic uraemic and normal subjects. *Brit. J. clin. Pharmacol., 2*:339–343.

Maren, T. H. (1967): Carbonic anhydrase: chemistry, physiology, and inhibition. *Physiol. Rev., 47*:595–781.

Milne, M. D., Schribner, B. H., and Crawford, M. A. (1958): Nonionic diffusion and the excretion of weak acids and bases. *Am. J. Med., 24*:709–729.

Morgan, T., Tadokoro, M., Martin, D., and Berliner, R. W. (1970): Effect of furosemide on Na^+ and K^+ transport studied by microperfusion of the rat nephron. *Am. J. Physiol., 218*:292–297.

Mudge, G. H. (1975): Diuretics and other agents employed in the mobilization of edema fluid. *In* L. S. Goodman and A. Gilman (eds.): *The Pharmacological Basis of Therapeutics*. 5th ed. New York, Macmillan, pp. 817–847.

Mussche, M. M., Belpaire, F. M., and Bogaert, M. G. (1975): Plasma protein binding of phenylbutazone during recovery from acute renal failure. *Europ. J. clin. Pharmacol., 9*:69–71.

Muth, R. G. (1971): Furosemide in severe renal insufficiency. *Postgrad. Med., 47*:21–25.

Nielsen, P., and Rasmussen, F. (1976): Elimination of trimethoprim, sulfadoxine and their metabolites in goats. *Acta Pharmacol. Toxicol., 38*:104–112.

O'Connell, J. M. B., Romeo, J. A., and Mudge, G. H. (1962): Renal tubular secretion of creatinine in the dog. *Am. J. Physiol., 203*:985–990.

Odar-Cederlöf, I., and Borga, O. (1974): Kinetics of diphenylhydantoin in uraemic patients: Consequences of decreased plasma protein binding. *Europ. J. clin. Pharmacol., 7*:31–37.

Olsen, G. D., Bennett, W. M., and Porter, G. A. (1975): Morphine and phenytoin binding to plasma protein in renal and hepatic failure. *Clin. Pharmacol. Ther., 17*:677–684.

O'Malley, K., Velasco, M., Pruitt, A., and McNay, J. L. (1975): Decreased plasma protein binding of diazoxide in uremia. *Clin. Pharmacol. Ther., 18*:53–58.

Pitts, R. F. (1968): *Physiology of the Kidney and Body Fluids*. 2nd Ed. Chicago, Year Book Medical Publishers.

Poulsen, E. (1957): Renal clearance in the cow. Copenhagen, Royal Veterinary and Agricultural College, Yearbook, pp. 97–126.

Preuss, H. G., Massry, S. G., Maher, J. F., Gilliece, M., and Schreiner, G. E. (1966): Effects of uremic sera on renal tubular *p*-aminohippurate transport. *Nephron, 3*:265–273.

Rane, A., Lunde, P. K. M., Jalling, B., Yaffee, S. J., and Sjoqvist, F. (1971): Plasma protein binding of diphenylhydantoin in normal and hyperbilirubinemic infants. *Pediat. Pharmacol. Ther., 78*:877–882.

Rasmussen, F. (1964): Salivary excretion of sulfonamides and barbiturates by cows and goats. *Acta Pharmacol. Toxicol., 21*:11–19.

Reidenberg, M. M. (1971): *Renal Function and Drug Action*. Philadelphia, W. B. Saunders Company.

Reidenberg, M. M., and Affrime, M. (1973): Influence of disease on binding of drugs to plasma proteins. *Ann. N.Y. Acad. Sci., 226*:115–126.

Reidenberg, M. M., James, M., and Dring, L. G. (1972): The rate of procaine hydrolysis in serum of normal subjects and diseased patients. *Clin. Pharmacol. Ther., 13*:279–284.

Reidenberg, M. M., Kostenbauder, H., and Adams, W. (1969): The rate of drug metabolism in obese volunteers before and during starvation and in azotemic patients. *Metabolism, 18*:209–213.

Reidenberg, M. M., Odar-Cederlöf, I., von Bahr, C., Borga, O., and Sjöqvist, F. (1971): Protein binding of diphenylhydantoin and desmethylimipramine in plasma from patients with poor renal function. *N. Engl. J. Med., 285*:264–267.

Reubi, F. C., and Coltier, P. T. (1961): Effects of reduced glomerular filtration rate on responsiveness to chlorothiazide and mercurial diuretics. *Circulation, 23*:200–210.

Richards, R. K., Taylor, J. D., and Kueter, K. E. (1953): Effect of nephrectomy on the duration of sleep following administration of thiopental and hexobarbital. *J. Pharmacol. exp. Ther., 108*:461–473.

Rose, J. H., Pruitt, A. W., and McNay, J. L. (1976): Effect of experimental azotemia on renal clearance of furosemide in the dog. *J. Pharmacol. exp. Ther., 196*:238–247.

Sachs, J., Geer, T., Noell, P., and Kunin, C. M. (1968): Effect of renal function on urinary recovery of orally administered nitrofurantoin. *N. Engl. J. Med., 278*:1032–1035.

Smith, H. W. (1951): *The Kidney: Structure and Function in Health and Disease.* New York, Oxford University Press.

Smith, H. W. (1956): *Principles of Renal Physiology.* New York, Oxford University Press.

Smith, W. M., Damato, A. N., Galluzzi, N. S., Garfield, C. F., Hanowell, E. G., Shinson, W. M., Thurm, R. H., Walsh, J. J., and Bromer, L. (1964): The evaluation of antihypertensive therapy: cooperative clinical trial method. *Ann. intern. Med., 61*:829–846.

Smith, W. M., Thurm, R. H., and Bromer, L. A. (1969): Comparative evaluation of Rauwolfia whole root and reserpine. *Clin. Pharmacol. Ther., 10*:338–343.

Soberman, R., Brodie, B. B., Levy, B. B., Axelrod, J., Hollander, V., and Steele, J. M. (1949): The use of antipyrine in the measurement of total body water in man. *J. Biol. Chem., 179*:31–42.

Swanson, R. E., and Hakim, A. A. (1962): Stop-flow analysis of creatinine excretion in the dog. *Am. J. Physiol., 203*:980–984.

Thaysen, J. H., and Schwartz, I. L. (1953): The permeability of human sweat glands to a series of sulfonamide compounds. *J. exp. Med., 98*:261–268.

Tozer, T. N. (1974): Nomogram for modification of dosage regimens in patients with chronic renal function impairment. *J. pharmacokinet. Biopharm., 2*:13–28.

Weiner, I. M., and Mudge, G. H. (1964): Renal tubular mechanisms for excretion of organic acids and bases. *Am. J. Med., 36*:743–762.

Welch, R. M., DeAngelis, R. L., Wingfield, M., and Farmer, T. W. (1975): Elimination of antipyrine from saliva as a measure of metabolism in man. *Clin. Pharmacol. Ther., 18*:249–258.

Whelton, A., and Walker, W. G. (1974): Intrarenal antibiotic distribution in health and disease [editorial]. *Kidney Internat., 6*:131–137.

Whelton, A., Carter, G. G., Bryant, H. H., Porteous, L. A., and Walker, W. G. (1973): Carbenicillin concentrations in normal and diseased kidneys. A therapeutic consideration. *Ann. intern. Med., 78*:659–662.

Whelton, A., Nightingale, S. D., Carter, G. G., Gordon, L. S., Bryant, H. H., and Walker, W. G. (1975): Pharmacokinetic characteristics of doxycycline accumulation in normal and severely diseased kidneys. *J. infect. Dis., 132*:467–471.

Whelton, A., Sapir, D. G., Carter, G. G., Garth, M. A., and Walker, W. G. (1972): Intrarenal distribution of ampicillin in the normal and diseased human kidney. *J. infect. Dis., 125*:466–470.

Whelton, A., Sapir, D. G., Carter, G. G., Kramer, J., and Walker, W. G. (1971): Intrarenal distribution of penicillin, cephalothin, ampicillin and oxytetracycline during varied states of hydration. *J. Pharmacol. exp. Ther., 179*:419–428.

Whelton, A., Schach von Wittenau, M., Twomey, T. M., Walker, W. G., and Bianchine, J. R. (1974): Doxycycline pharmacokinetics in the absence of renal function. *Kidney Internat., 5*:365–371.

Williams, R. T. (1971): Species variations in drug biotransformations. *In* B. N. LaDu, H. G. Mandel and E. L. Way (eds.): *Fundamentals of Drug Metabolism and Drug Disposition.* Baltimore, Williams & Wilkins, pp. 187–205.

Wilson, W. E. C., Kirkpatrick, C. H., and Talmage, D. W. (1965): Suppression of immunologic responsiveness in uremia. *Ann. intern. Med., 62*:1–14.

6

Principles of Pharmacokinetics

INTRODUCTION

Pharmacokinetics is defined as the mathematical description of concentration changes of drugs within the body. A common approach to studying the pharmacokinetic behavior of drugs is to depict the body as a system of distribution compartments (Riegelman et al., 1968a). In many instances these compartments, which are mathematical entities, have no physiological meaning but are useful in describing the disposition kinetics of a drug. The "two-compartment open model" (Fig. 6–1) adequately describes the disposition of many drugs in humans and animals. It is assumed that a drug entering the body distributes instantaneously and homogeneously into a space termed the central compartment, which consists of the blood and other readily accessible tissues and fluids. For many drugs the central compartment probably consists of the blood plasma and the extracellular fluid of highly perfused organs, such as the lungs, liver, heart and kidneys. Distribution into the remainder of the available body space, or peripheral compartment, takes place more slowly. The peripheral (or tissue) compartment may be considered to consist of less well-perfused tissues, such as muscle, skin and body fat. The apparent volume of the central and peripheral compartments for each drug depends on the characteristics of blood flow to each component tissue, on the drug's ability to enter these tissues from the circulation and on the extent of tissue binding. Compartments for drug distribution can have apparent volumes in

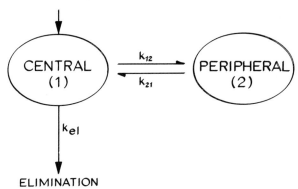

ELIMINATION

Figure 6–1 Schematic diagram of the two-compartment open model. The dose of drug is introduced into the central compartment, where it distributes instantaneously. Distribution between central and peripheral compartments takes place more slowly; k_{12} and k_{21} are first-order rate constants for drug transfer between the two compartments. Elimination, which comprises biotransformation and excretion, is assumed to occur exclusively from the central compartment; k_{el} is the first-order rate constant for drug elimination from the central compartment.

excess of their true volumes because of binding to tissue constituents (e.g., proteins).

The two-compartment model specifies that drugs enter the system only via the central compartment and that elimination (i.e., biotransformation and excretion) takes place exclusively from the central compartment. The distribution and elimination processes associated with the model are assumed to follow first-order kinetics. Accordingly, the rate at which a drug is removed from a compartment is proportional to the drug concentration in it. The purpose of pharmacokinetics is to study the time course of drug and metabolite concentrations and amounts in various body fluids, tissues and excreta, and to construct suitable models to interpret such data (Wagner, 1968a).

PRINCIPLES OF PHARMACOKINETIC ANALYSIS

Pharmacokinetic principles relate specifically to the variation with time of drug concentration, particularly in the blood plasma or serum. By extrapolation, they may be interpreted in terms of drug effect. The simplest method of drug administration for pharmacokinetic analysis is the rapid injection of a single dose directly into the bloodstream (an intravenous bolus). Assuming instantaneous distribution throughout the central compartment, the rate of decrease in plasma concentration of the drug may be written:

$$-\frac{dC_P}{dt} = (k_{12} + k_{el})C_P - k_{21}C_T \qquad \textbf{Equation 6 • 1}$$

where C_P is the concentration of drug in plasma and C_T is the drug concentration in the distribution fluids (tissues) at time t. Solution of this differential equation yields the biexponential expression:

$$C_P = Ae^{-\alpha t} + Be^{-\beta t} \qquad \textbf{Equation 6 • 2}$$

in which the coefficients A and B are "intercept" terms with dimensions of concentration (μg/ml), α and β are the distribution and elimination rate constants, respectively, which are expressed in units of reciprocal time (min^{-1}), and e represents the base of the natural logarithm. The

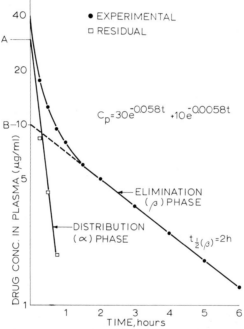

Figure 6–2 Semilogarithmic graph depicting the time course of drug in the plasma after intravenous administration of a single dose (10 mg/kg). The disposition curve is described by the biexponential expression:

$$C_P = 30e^{-0.058t} + 10e^{-0.0058t}$$

where C_P is the concentration of the drug in plasma at time t. The initial plasma drug concentration ($C_P^0 = 40$ μg/ml) is the sum of A and B. The half-life of the drug is defined as:

$$t_{1/2(\beta)} = \frac{ln\ 2}{\beta} = \frac{0.693}{\beta}$$

where β (0.0058 min $^{-1}$) is the negative value of the slope of the linear terminal portion (elimination phase) of the disposition curve.

mathematical expression in Equation 6·2 frequently describes the semilogarithmic graph of the decline of drug concentration in the plasma as a function of time after intravenous administration of a single dose of the drug (Fig. 6–2). The initial steep decline in plasma drug concentration is due mainly to distribution (by diffusion) of the drug from the central to peripheral (tissue) compartment. Once apparent (pseudo-) distribution equilibrium is established, the rate of decline in plasma drug concentration is reduced and determined mainly by irreversible elimination of drug from the central compartment, appropriately termed the "beta" or "elimination" phase (Fig. 6–3). This linear portion of the curve has a slope which may be defined as $-\beta/2.303$ and an extrapolated zero-time intercept, B, expressed in units of concentration. Resolving the biexponential drug

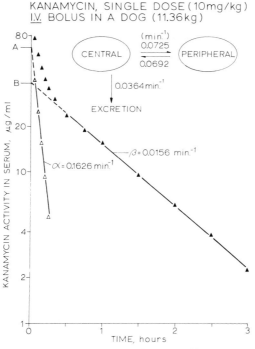

Figure 6–3 Analysis of the disposition kinetics of kanamycin in a dog given a single intravenous dose (10 mg/kg) of kanamycin sulfate (50 mg/ml). The elimination phase is represented by a least squares linear regression line, based on measured activity of kanamycin in serum samples (▲) between 0.5 and 3 hours after drug administration. The regression line which represents distribution phase is based on calculated data points (△), which were obtained by the feathering technique. Note the much smaller value of β compared to α. Inset is a schematic representation of the two-compartment open model; values of the individual rate constants (microconstants) associated with the model are given.

disposition curve into its two components by the method of residuals yields a second linear segment, called the "alpha" or "distribution" phase, with a slope equal to $-\alpha/2.303$ and a zero-time intercept of A (Gibaldi et al., 1969). If the ordinate of the semilogarithmic graph were in natural logarithms (base e) the slopes of the two exponential components of the disposition curve would be simply $-\alpha$ and $-\beta$. The sum of A and B gives the drug concentration in the plasma immediately following intravenous injection ($C^0{}_p$). The apparent volume of the central compartment, V_c, is estimated by the expression:

$$V_c = \frac{\text{Dose}_{(\text{I.V.})}}{C^0{}_P}$$

Equation 6 • 3

In drug disposition studies, one calculates the coefficients A and B and the rate constants α and β from the plasma drug concentration–time

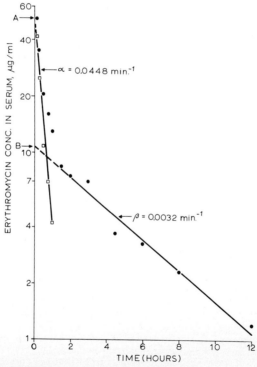

Figure 6–4 The decline of erythromycin concentration in serum (log scale) with time (linear scale) following intravenous injection of a single dose (12.5 mg/kg) of the drug to a cow. Distribution and elimination phases of erythromycin disposition are represented by least squares regression lines. Constants A and B are the zero-time intercepts of distribution and elimination phases, respectively (see Table 6–1). (From Baggot, J. D., and Gingerich, D. A. [1976]: *Res. vet. Sci.*, 21:318–323.)

data. These experimental constants are "hybrid" pharmacokinetic parameters. A semilogarithmic graph of the experimental data provides an idea of the time at which apparent distribution equilibrium is established. Iterative least squares linear regression lines should be used to derive the values for B and β which best fit the terminal exponential phase of the disposition curve. Values for A and α, which describe the distribution component of the disposition curve, should be obtained by computing a least squares linear regression line for the residual data points obtained by calculation from the initial portion of the semilogarithmic graph by the method of residuals or feathering technique (Figs. 6–4, 6–5 and 6–6). The residual data points, which represent the distribution phase, are obtained by subtracting the extrap-

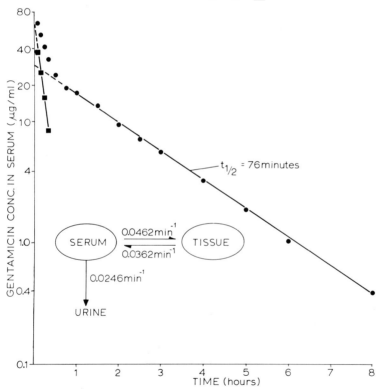

Figure 6–5 Serum levels of gentamicin (•) following administration of a single intravenous dose (10 mg/kg) to a dog. The least squares linear regression line, which represents distribution phase of gentamicin disposition, was based on calculated data points (■). Gentamicin is eliminated by urinary excretion. The data were analyzed according to a two-compartment open model (inset). Values of kinetic constants are given in Table 6–1.

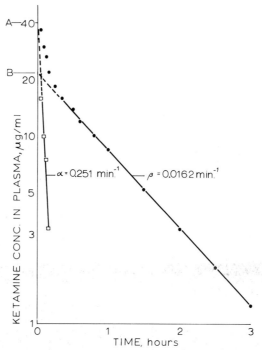

Figure 6-6 Semilogarithmic plot of ketamine concentration in plasma versus time after administration of a single dose of ketamine hydrochloride (25 mg/kg) as an intravenous bolus to a cat (3.24 kg body weight). The biexponential decline of plasma drug concentration indicates that ketamine confers two-compartment model characteristics on the body. Values of kinetic constants are given in Table 6-1. (From Baggot, J. D., and Blake, J. W. [1976]: *Arch. int. Pharmacodyn. Thér.*, 220:115–124.)

olated portion of the β phase from the experimental data. The need to determine the most accurate equation to describe the disposition curve is crucial. Perhaps the best approach is to fit the entire plasma level-time curve by means of a digital computer program, which provides a nonlinear regression analysis of the curve (Fig. 6-7).

The plasma drug concentration–time profile is important because it represents the only relevant information that can be accurately measured for most drugs. In other words, it is the only reliable source of quantifiable experimental data. The experimental constants (A, B, α and β) are used to calculate the actual pharmacokinetic rate constants associated with the two-compartment open model (k_{12}, k_{21}, k_{el}). Two sets of equations for obtaining values of the microconstants are given:

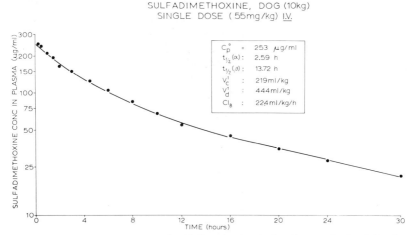

SULFADIMETHOXINE, DOG (10kg)
SINGLE DOSE (55mg/kg) I.V.

C_p°	253 $\mu g/ml$
$t_{1/2}(\alpha)$:	2.59 h
$t_{1/2}(\beta)$:	13.72 h
V_c^1 :	219ml/kg
V_d^1 :	444ml/kg
Cl_B :	224ml/kg/h

Figure 6–7 Concentrations of sulfadimethoxine in the plasma of a dog following the intravenous injection of a single dose (55 mg/kg). The curve is based on a non-linear regression analysis of the data, which were interpreted as conferring two-compartment model characteristics on the body.

$$k_{21} = A^1\beta + B^1\alpha$$

$$k_{21} = \frac{A\beta + B\alpha}{A + B}$$

Equation 6 • 4

where $A^1 = A/C^0_p$, $B^1 = B/C^0_p$

$$k_{el} = \frac{1}{(A^1/\alpha + B^1/\beta)}$$

$$A + B = C^0_P$$

$$k_{el} = \frac{\alpha\beta}{k_{21}}$$

Equation 6 • 5

$$k_{12} = \frac{A^1 B^1 (\beta - \alpha)^2}{k_{21}}$$

$$k_{12} = \alpha + \beta - k_{21} - k_{el}$$

Equation 6 • 6

Determination of the microconstants permits an assessment of the relative contribution of distribution and elimination processes (which may be altered in disease states) to the concentration–time profile of a drug.

In evaluating data that are best described by a two-compartment open model, several parameters can be classified as "hybrid" in that their values change disproportionately with the magnitude of the elimination rate constant (k_{el}). These parameters are: α, β, A, B, $t_{1/2(\beta)}$, f_c, $V_{d(\beta)}$, $V_{d(area)}$, and $V_{d(B)}$ (Jusko and Gibaldi, 1972). The hybrid parameters should not be used individually as a direct or sole measure of a change in drug elimination or distribution.

Values of the kinetic parameters which describe the disposition of ketamine in a cat, gentamicin in a dog and erythromycin in a cow are given in Table 6–1. The data presented in this table are related to the graphs in Figures 6–4, 6–5 and 6–6. The technique for pharmacokinetic analysis of plasma concentration versus time data is similar for any class of drug given by the intravenous route and is applicable to all species of animals. The extent of individual variation in values of the kinetic parameters describing disposition of a drug depends on the uniformity, age and state of health of the group of animals, as well as on the fate of the compound. The disposition kinetics of gentamicin in normal beagles given a single intravenous dose (10 mg/kg) of gentamicin sulfate (Gentocin, 50 mg/ml) provide an example of individual variation found among normal dogs for a drug eliminated by renal excretion (Table 6–2). The fate of sulfadimethoxine has been described in humans and various species of animals (Bridges et al., 1968). In dogs the drug is excreted mainly unchanged in the urine, which also contains small amounts of the N^1- and N^4-glucuronide derivatives. The disposition kinetics of sulfadimethoxine in beagles ($n = 6$) following intravenous injection of a single dose (55 mg/kg) show the degree of individual variation in pharmacokinetic parameters

Table 6–1 PHARMACOKINETIC PARAMETERS WHICH DESCRIBE DISPOSITION OF VARIOUS DRUGS FOLLOWING ADMINISTRATION OF A SINGLE INTRAVENOUS DOSE

Kinetic Parameter	Units of Measurement	Erythromycin (Cow)	Gentamicin (Dog)	Ketamine (Cat)
C^0_P	μg/ml	62.5	93.0	62.5
A	μg/ml	51.8	64.6	40.6
α	min^{-1}	0.0448	0.0979	0.2510
$t_{1/2(\alpha)}$	min	15.5	7.1	2.76
B	μg/ml	10.7	28.4	21.9
β	min^{-1}	0.0032	0.0091	0.0162
$t_{1/2(\beta)}$	min	216.6	76.3	42.8
k_{12}	min^{-1}	0.0236	0.0462	0.1272
k_{21}	min^{-1}	0.0104	0.0362	0.0984
k_{el}	min^{-1}	0.0139	0.0246	0.0413
V'_c	liter/kg	0.200	0.107	0.400
$V'_{d(area)}$	liter/kg	0.860	0.291	1.151
Cl_B	ml/kg/min	2.72	2.64	18.5
Dose	mg/kg	12.5	10.0	25.0
Body weight	kg	568	10.0	3.24
Semilogarithmic graph		Figure 6–4	Figure 6–5	Figure 6–6

Table 6-2 DISPOSITION KINETICS OF GENTAMICIN IN NORMAL BEAGLES ($n = 7$) AFTER INTRAVENOUS ADMINISTRATION OF A SINGLE DOSE (10 MG/KG) OF GENTAMICIN SULFATE (GENTOCIN, 50 MG/ML)

Kinetic Parameter	Units	Mean ± S.D.	Median (Range)
C^0_P	μg/ml	92.7 ± 18.3	93.0(65.9–112.7)
A	μg/ml	67.4 ± 15.8	69.7(40.1–86.8)
α	min^{-1}	0.0925 ± 0.0162	0.0969(0.0648–0.1100)
$t_{1/2(\alpha)}$	min	7.7 ± 1.5	7.2(6.3–10.7)
B	μg/ml	25.4 ± 9.4	25.9(13.1–42.1)
β	min^{-1}	0.0092 ± 0.0006	0.0091(0.0082–0.0101)
$t_{1/2(\beta)}$	min	75.6 ± 4.9	75.8(68.9–84.2)
k_{12}	min^{-1}	0.0423 ± 0.0116	0.0433(0.0227–0.0558)
k_{21}	min^{-1}	0.0319 ± 0.0075	0.0323(0.0182–0.0420)
k_{el}	min^{-1}	0.0276 ± 0.0059	0.0290(0.0204–0.0358)
V'_c	ml/kg	111 ± 25	107(85–152)
$V'_{d(area)}$	ml/kg	335 ± 94.5	305(207–466)
$V'_{d(B)}$	ml/kg	448 ± 182	386(238–762)
Cl_B	ml/kg/min	2.94 ± 0.67	2.86(1.83–3.84)
$C_{P(8\ hr)}$	μg/ml	0.33 ± 0.15	0.31(0.16–0.62)
Body weight	kg	9.36 ± 0.90	9.54(8.18–10.65)
Renal Function:			
GFR	ml/kg/min	5.43 ± 0.78	5.22(4.55–6.63)
ERPF	ml/kg/min	16.09 ± 3.71	15.26(12.32–21.97)

Renal function was measured by single intravenous injection technique, using ^{125}I-iothalamate and ^{131}I-iodohippurate, five days before administration of gentamicin.

Table 6-3 DISPOSITION KINETICS OF SULFADIMETHOXINE IN BEAGLES ($n = 6$) AFTER ADMINISTRATION OF A SINGLE INTRAVENOUS DOSE (55 MG/KG) OF SULFADIMETHOXINE FOR INJECTION (BACTROVET, 10 PER CENT)

Kinetic Parameter	Units	Mean ± S.D.	Median (Range)
C^0_P	μg/ml	266.5 ± 46.0	257(212–344)
A	μg/ml	152.4 ± 43.5	151.5(90.4–212.5)
$t_{1/2(\alpha)}$	hours	2.5 ± 0.45	2.36(2.06–3.35)
B	μg/ml	114.0 ± 22.0	105(89.4–149.3)
$t_{1/2(\beta)}$	hours	13.2 ± 2.2	13.1(9.7–16.5)
k_{12}	hour^{-1}	0.083 ± 0.019	0.092(0.051–0.097)
k_{21}	hour^{-1}	0.155 ± 0.034	0.153(0.108–0.209)
k_{el}	hour^{-1}	0.100 ± 0.021	0.098(0.078–0.139)
V'_c	ml/kg	211 ± 34	214(160–259)
$V'_{d(area)}$	ml/kg	405 ± 63	410(312–502)
Cl_B	ml/kg/hour	21.4 ± 2.4	21.7(17.8–24.6)
$C_{P(24\ hr)}$	μg/ml	33 ± 7	31.5(25–42)
Body weight	kg	9.92 ± 0.87	9.75(9.0–11.0)

for a long-acting compound (Table 6–3). Variations in elimination kinetics of extensively metabolized drugs are usually greater between herbivorous and carnivorous species, and between ruminant animals and horses and between dogs and cats, than individual variations among animals within a single species. One would expect to find a higher degree of individual variation in drug disposition among diseased animals as a result of fever, dehydration, impaired renal function, uremia, hypoproteinemia, and so forth, than among normal animals.

Critical features of a disposition study are the design of the *in vivo* experiment (state of health of the animal, blood sampling schedule, knowledge of the fate and pharmacological effects of the drug), handling and storage of the blood samples and the analytical method for quantitative determination of the drug. It is essential that the drug assay method be sensitive and specific. One should know whether the total or the free drug in plasma is being measured, and the extent of plasma protein binding should be determined at therapeutic concentrations of the drug. This information is necessary for interpretation of the data generated in a drug disposition study. Although the usual number of experimental subjects is at least six animals, pharmacokinetic analysis of the data should be performed for each individual animal. It is exceedingly difficult, if not impossible, to determine if a given set of whole blood, plasma or serum concentrations of a drug measured after a single dose is best described by a classical linear or nonlinear mathematical model. The problem is even more difficult with urinary data. Obtaining data after only one or two doses of a drug usually supplies insufficient information to deduce the appropriate model. It is not uncommon for known nonlinear data to appear to be linear when only one dose of a drug is studied (Wagner, 1973).

When equilibration of a drug between the central and peripheral compartments is very rapid relative to the rate of elimination ($k_{12} + k_{21} \gg k_{el}$), the disposition kinetics of the drug may be adequately described by assuming the body to behave as a single homogeneous distribution compartment—i.e., the one-compartment open model. The one-compartment model assumes that any changes that occur in the plasma reflect quantitatively changes occurring in tissue drug levels. This does not necessarily imply that the drug concentrations in all body tissues at any given time are the same. The decrease in plasma concentration of the drug as a function of time may be described mathematically by the monoexponential expression:

$$C_P = Be^{-\beta t}$$ **Equation 6 • 7**

where B is the zero-time intercept of the least squares linear regression line and β is the overall elimination rate constant, being the negative value of the slope of the line. The value of the coefficient B is an estimate of the initial drug concentration in plasma based on instantaneous attainment of distribution equilibrium. Drugs whose disposition kinetics can be adequately described by the one-compartment open model include amphetamine (Baggot and Davis, 1973), chloramphenicol (Davis et al., 1972) and quinidine (Neff et al., 1972) in domestic animals. A two-compartment open model best describes the disposition of quinidine in humans (Ueda et al., 1976).

To completely describe the disposition kinetics of some drugs it may be necessary to analyze the data according to a three-compartment open model. The mathematical expression which describes the plasma drug concentration–time profile following intravenous administration of a single dose is:

$$C_p = Pe^{-\pi t} + Ae^{-\alpha t} + Be^{-\beta t} \qquad \textbf{Equation 6 • 8}$$

Values of P, A, B, π, α and β can be estimated from the semilogarithmic plot of plasma drug concentration versus time, which is a triexponential curve. Although such estimates can be made employing the method of residuals, the best method to determine these terms is to fit the curve by nonlinear least squares regression analysis. Once the experimental constants $(P, A, B, \pi, \alpha$ and $\beta)$ are known, the apparent volume of the central compartment (V_c) and the individual rate constants associated with the three-compartment open model $(k_{12}, k_{21}, k_{13}, k_{31},$ and $k_{el})$ can be calculated (Gibaldi and Perrier, 1975). The number of distribution compartments is equal to the number of exponential expressions required to describe drug disposition. A three-compartment open model best describes disposition of digoxin (Kramer et al., 1974), pentazocine (Vaughan and Beckett, 1974) and diazepam (Kaplan et al., 1973) in humans, sulfadimethoxine in bovine animals (Boxenbaum and Kaplan, 1975), naloxone in dogs (Sams et al., 1976 [personal communication]) and oxytetracycline in dogs and horses. A semilogarithmic plot of the experimental oxytetracycline serum concentrations obtained following intravenous administration of a single dose (5 mg/kg) to a dog and the computer simulated curve are shown in Figure 6–8. The pharmacokinetic parameters that describe disposition of the antibiotic in normal dogs are given in Table 6–4. The decline in serum oxytetracycline activity with time after intravenous injection of a single dose (4.4 mg/kg) in horses is best described by a three-compartment open model, but a two-compartment model adequately describes the experimental data for some individuals (Figs. 6–9 and 6–10).

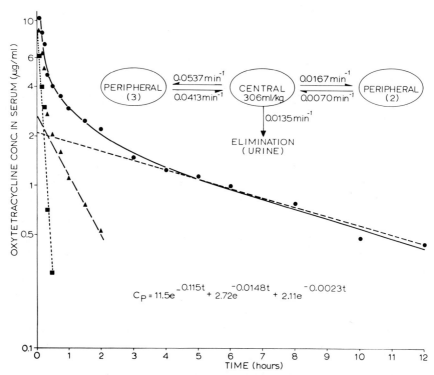

OXYTETRACYCLINE, DOG (10.42kg)
SINGLE DOSE (5mg/kg) I.V.

$$C_P = 11.5e^{-0.115t} + 2.72e^{-0.0148t} + 2.11e^{-0.0023t}$$

Figure 6–8 Analysis of the disposition kinetics of oxytetracycline in a dog given a single intravenous dose. Closed circles (•) represent the measured serum concentrations (activity) of the antibiotic; other data points were calculated by the method of residuals. The simulated curve (solid line) is based on a nonlinear regression analysis of the data, which confer three-compartment model characteristics (inset) on the body. The triexponential equation which describes the disposition curve is given.

Table 6–4 PHARMACOKINETIC PARAMETERS DESCRIBING DISPOSITION OF OXYTETRACYCLINE IN DOGS (n = 6) AFTER INTRAVENOUS INJECTION OF A SINGLE DOSE (5 MG/KG)

Kinetic Parameter	Units	Mean ± S.D.
C^0_P	μg/ml	21.36 ± 4.55
P	μg/ml	16.77 ± 4.18
π	min⁻¹	0.124 ± 0.030
A	μg/ml	2.85 ± 0.59
α	min⁻¹	0.0125 ± 0.0013
B	μg/ml	1.75 ± 0.57
β	min⁻¹	0.0020 ± 0.0005
$t_{1/2(\beta)}$	min	360 ± 90
V'_c	ml/kg	242.5 ± 48.2
$V'_{d(area)}$	ml/kg	2096 ± 422
$V'_{d(B)}$	ml/kg	3100 ± 906
Cl_B	ml/kg/min	4.23 ± 1.29
k_{12}	min⁻¹	0.0178 ± 0.0019
k_{21}	min⁻¹	0.0053 ± 0.0011
k_{13}	min⁻¹	0.0637 ± 0.0223
k_{31}	min⁻¹	0.0344 ± 0.0069
k_{el}	min⁻¹	0.0178 ± 0.0060
$C_{P(8\ hr)}$	μg/ml	0.72 ± 0.30
Body weight	kg	10.52 ± 0.51

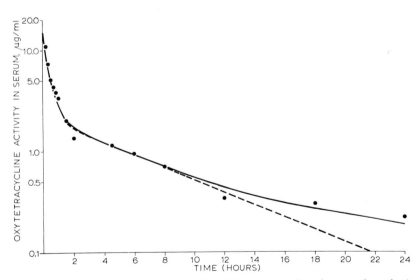

Figure 6–9 Decline in serum oxytetracycline activity, plotted on semilogarthmic graph paper, after intravenous administration of a single dose (4.4 mg/kg) to a standardbred mare (457 kg body weight). Two-compartment (– – –) and three-compartment (——) model curves obtained by nonlinear least squares regression analysis of the data are given. Based on fit of the curves to the data, the drug confers the characteristics of a three-compartment model on the body.

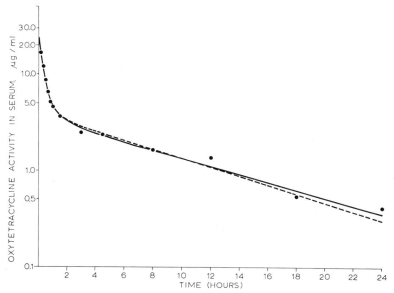

Figure 6–10 The time course of oxytetracycline activity in serum of a standard-bred mare (437 kg body weight) given a single intravenous dose (4.4 mg/kg). Comparison of two-compartment (− − −) and three-compartment (——) model curves shows that the data can be adequately described by a biexponential expression.

Significance of the Overall Elimination Rate Constant

The overall elimination rate constant (β) is probably the most important functional pharmacokinetic parameter in a drug disposition study. It is equal to the negative value of the slope of the linear terminal phase of the plot $ln\ C_p$ versus time. The overall elimination rate constant is a component of equations used to calculate half-life, volume of distribution (by the area method), body clearance, microconstants of multicompartment (two or more) models, and dosage intervals of multiple dose regimens. It is also essential in determining infusion rates for drugs and the absorption rate constants following drug administration by nonintravascular routes. The time it takes to reach plasma steady-state level of a drug when a fixed dose is given at constant intervals is related to the magnitude of β. Another possible application for this hybrid constant is in predicting withdrawal periods for drug products in residue studies (Mercer et al., 1977). This application is based on the assumption (which must be verified experimentally) that the semilogarithmic plots of drug disappearance from plasma (or serum) and tissues (e.g., liver, skeletal muscle, kidney, etc.) have the same slope.

The half-time for elimination of a drug is called the (biological) half-life, which is defined as the time required for the body to eliminate one-half of the particular drug. The assumption is made that once distribution equilibrium has been established the ratio of the drug in peripheral-to-central compartments remains constant. The terms biological and plasma (or serum) half-life, as defined here, are synonymous, and the parameter will hereafter be referred to simply as the "half-life." The half-life value is obtained from the expression:

$$t_{1/2} = \frac{0.693}{\beta}$$
        Equation 6 • 9

where β is the overall elimination rate constant, and $t_{1/2}$ is expressed in units of time (minutes or hours). A large value of β, corresponding to a short half-life, indicates rapid elimination. The rate of drug elimination may be influenced by extensive binding to plasma proteins, the rates of various metabolic pathways (hepatic microsomal oxidation predominates for lipid-soluble compounds) and the efficiency of excretion processes (particularly glomerular filtration). Each time an interval equal to 1 half-life of a drug elapses, 50 per cent of the drug that was present in the body at the beginning of that interval has been eliminated. Exponential (first-order) elimination implies that a constant fraction of drug contained in the body is eliminated per unit of time. The half-life values of the majority of drugs that are used as therapeutic agents in humans and domestic animals are independent of the dose administered, since their overall elimination obeys first-order kinetics. Furthermore, the half-life of a drug that is eliminated exponentially is independent of the route of administration. However, the intravenous injection of a single dose of drug is the only satisfactory procedure for determining the half-life value. The apparent overall elimination rate constant (β^1), which is obtained from the slope of the linear terminal phase of the semilogarithmic graph of plasma drug concentration versus time after other than intravenous (e.g., oral, S.C., I.M.) administration of a drug product, may be influenced by the rate of absorption (Byron and Notari, 1976).

Dose-Dependent Elimination

Biotransformation reactions, carrier-mediated transport (including renal and biliary secretion) and protein binding of drugs are saturable processes. The concentrations of most drugs at sites of elimination following administration of therapeutic doses are within the capacity of the particular systems, so that first-order kinetics are obeyed. Traditionally, it has been assumed that the kinetics of elimination of alcohol from the blood of animals and humans can be described as zero-order—i.e., independent of the blood concentration (above about 2 to 3 mM or 0.09 to 0.14 mg/ml). Some investigators make this assumption simply because part of the blood alcohol concentration–time curve appears to be linear, whereas others believe that liver alcohol dehydrogenase is saturated at low concentrations of alcohol (Hawkins and Kalant, 1972). Recently, Wagner and co-workers (1976) demonstrated that zero-order kinetics are inappropriate for describing the elimination of alcohol in humans. The rate of metabolism of alcohol is described more accurately by the V_{max} and K_m values and the Michaelis-Menten equation:

$$-\frac{dC}{dt} = \frac{V_{max} \cdot C}{(K_m + C)} \qquad \textbf{Equation 6 • 10}$$

where C is the blood alcohol concentration at time t, K_m is the Michaelis constant, and V_{max} is the maximum velocity. The metabolism of salicylic acid in humans (Levy, 1965) is an example of a saturable process. Dose-dependent kinetics are also important when bishydroxycoumarin (Nagashima et al., 1968), phenylbutazone (Burns et al., 1953) and phenytoin (Arnold and Gerber, 1970) are given to humans. The half-life of salicylate is dose-dependent in cats (Yeary and Swanson, 1973) and phenylbutazone elimination follows zero-order kinetics in dogs (Dayton et al., 1967) and horses (Piperno et al., 1968). An increase in dosage of such a drug results in a more prolonged half-life and a disproportionately greater accumulation of drug in the body. Zero-order elimination means that a constant amount of the drug in the body is eliminated per unit of time.* Suitable dosage regimens for drugs exhibiting dose-dependent kinetics in the therapeutic dose range defy easy calculation and are established by careful titration of drug levels in the patient (Levy, 1968).

Half-Life of a Drug

The half-life is a measure of the rate of drug elimination, being the time taken for the plasma (or serum) concentration of the drug to decline by 50 per cent during the elimination phase of the disposition curve (plasma drug concentration–time profile). Half-life is inversely

---

*Dose-dependent elimination is usually, but not always, the result of saturation of a drug-metabolizing enzyme system. Dependence of plasma quinine half-life upon dose was observed in dogs and attributed primarily to an increased apparent volume of distribution of the drug (Berlin et al., 1975).

related to the overall elimination rate constant, and the calculated value based on β ($t_{1/2} = 0.693/\beta$) is the most accurate (Gibaldi and Weintraub, 1971). An estimate of the half-life of a drug may be obtained graphically from a semilogarithmic plot of plasma drug concentration (on a logarithmic scale) versus time (on a linear scale) following intravenous administration of a single dose of the drug (Fig. 6–11). The half-life is found by measuring the time required for a given plasma level of the drug to decline by 50 per cent during the terminal exponential (β) phase of the curve. Elimination of the drug depicted in Figure 6–11 obeys first-order kinetics and the half-life is 1.5 hours. Knowledge of the half-life of a drug can be extremely useful in a

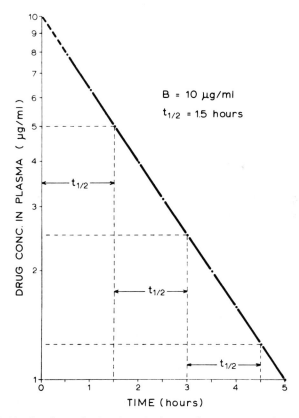

Figure 6–11 Semilogarithmic plot of plasma drug concentration versus time following administration of a single intravenous dose. The monoexponential decline corresponds to elimination (β) phase of the disposition curve and suggests that kinetics may be adequately described by the one-compartment open model. Graphical technique for estimating the half-life of a drug (1.5 hours for this drug) is illustrated. The half-life is the time required for the plasma drug concentration at any point on the straight line to decrease by one-half.

predictive sense, particularly with respect to the design of rational dosage regimens. On the premise that the distribution and elimination processes follow first-order kinetics, multiples of the half-life give a crude estimate of the fraction of original amount of drug remaining in the body at intervals after administration of a single dose or the last of a series of doses (Table 6–5).

The elimination of a drug can be based on measurements of cumulative drug excretion in the urine. When the drug is not metabolized and is excreted only in the urine, the amount of drug remaining in the body can be calculated directly from the total dose administered and the amount of drug excreted in the given interval:

Total dose administered − Amount excreted =   **Equation 6 • 11**

Quantity of drug remaining in the body (amount unexcreted)

When the fraction (or percentage) of drug as yet unexcreted is plotted (on a logarithmic scale) against time (on an arithmetic scale), a straight line will be obtained if first-order kinetics hold, from which the half-life can be obtained and the overall elimination rate constant computed (Nelson and O'Reilly, 1960). Obviously, if elimination processes other than renal excretion contribute significantly to removal of drug from the body, an apparent (rather than true) overall elimination rate constant is obtained by measuring cumulative excretion of unchanged drug in the urine. The apparent overall elimination rate constant reflects only the renal contribution to the overall elimination process. When a drug is metabolized as well as excreted unchanged in urine, the kinetics of its elimination can be interpolated from urinary excretion data, provided that the metabolites are excreted in the urine and can be quantitated. In this situation, the amount of

Table 6–5   ESTIMATION OF FRACTION OF ORIGINAL AMOUNT OF DRUG REMAINING IN THE BODY FROM NUMBER OF HALF-LIVES, ASSUMING FIRST-ORDER KINETICS

| Portion of Original Amount Remaining | | Time After Dosing |
FRACTION	PER CENT	(Multiples of $t_{1/2}$)
$1/2$	50	1
$1/4$	25	2
$1/8$	12.5	3
$1/16$	6.25	4
$1/32$	3.125	5
$1/64$	1.5625	6
$1/256$	0.3906	8
$1/1024$	0.097	10

drug unexcreted is equal to the difference between the total amount of unchanged drug plus its metabolites in urine and the difference between the amount of drug administered (dose) and the total amount of unchanged drug plus its metabolites in the urine.

The half-life, which is a measure of the overall rate of elimination, is influenced by all the factors which govern elimination. For compounds whose fate includes hepatic biotransformation and renal excretion, overall rate of elimination is determined by the activities of the particular metabolic reactions and the efficiency of renal excretion, the blood flow to the liver and kidneys and the fraction of the dose that is available to the sites of elimination. This latter parameter is determined by the extent of binding to plasma proteins and the magnitude of distribution. The half-life and principal process of elimination of some drugs in dogs are given in Table 6-6. Although a particular elimination process usually predominates (e.g., oxidation by hepatic microsomal enzymes, renal excretion by glomerular filtration), elimination of most drugs involves a combination of processes that occur simultaneously.

Superimposed on the numerous factors influencing the half-life of a drug in an individual animal are intra- and interspecies variations. Studies with the anti-inflammatory agent phenylbutazone pointed out the importance of species differences in drug metabolism (Burns et al., 1960). Significant differences in half-lives of several drugs, in particular those extensively metabolized, exist among species of domestic animals (Table 6-7). Ruminant animals appear to be endowed with highly efficient hepatic biotransformation mechanisms. One may hypothesize that interspecies variations are likely to exist in the half-lives of drugs eliminated mainly by biotransformation (lipid-soluble compounds), particularly when the metabolic process is mediated by the hepatic microsomal enzyme systems. Knowledge of whether the plasma levels of a drug or its metabolite(s), or both, correlate with the drug's pharmacological activity and toxicity in various animal species is highly important in determining the significance of species differences in rates and pathways of biotransformation. Interspecies variation in half-life is not so pronounced for drugs that are eliminated by excretion. When glomerular filtration is the principal mechanism of drug excretion, the half-life is usually shorter in dogs than in the herbivorous species of domestic animals. Elimination of kanamycin, an aminoglycoside antibiotic and polar compound, in dogs, horses and sheep given the same dose (10 mg/kg) by intravenous injection serves to illustrate this point (Fig. 6-12). Likewise, the half-life (mean ± S.D., $n = 5$) of oxytetracycline is of similar length in horses (10.5 ± 2.9 hours) and cows (9.12 ± 1.50 hours) and is considerably shorter in dogs (6.02 ± 1.5 hours, $n = 6$). Whether drug therapy should be initiated with a priming dose is related to the mechanism of action and

Table 6–6   HALF-LIFE VALUES AND PRINCIPAL PROCESS OF ELIMINATION OF DRUGS IN THE DOG

Drug	Half-Life (Hours)	Process(es) of Elimination
Penicillin G	0.5	E(r)
Kanamycin	0.9	E(r)
Gentamicin	1.25	E(r)
Tylosin	0.9	E(b + r) + M
Griseofulvin	0.8	M
Colistin methanesulfonate	1.4	
Trimethoprim	3.0	M
Chloramphenicol	4.2	M
Oxytetracycline	6.0	E(r)
Doxycycline	—	
Sulfisoxazole	4.5	E(r)
Sulfadimethoxine	13.2	E(r) + M
Pentazocine	0.4	M
Pethidine (meperidine)	0.9	M
Naloxone	1.5	M
Morphine	—	
Diazepam, N-desmethyldiazepam	—	
Clonazepam	5.4	M
Pentobarbitone	4.5	M
Amphetamine	4.5	M + E(r)
Methylphenidate, ritalinic acid	2.5 to 3.0	M + E(r)
Phenacetin	0.6	M
Acetaminophen	—	M
Salicylate	8.6	M
Seclazone	8.5	M
Phenylbutazone	3.0 to 8.0*	M
Oxyphenbutazone	1.7	M
Procainamide	2.0	E(r) + M
Quinidine	5.6	M
Propranolol, 4-hydroxypropranolol	0.6	M
Sotalol	4.8	E
Hydrocortisone	0.75	M
Cortisone	0.5	M
9α-F-Hydrocortisone	0.97	M
Prednisone	0.55	M
Prednisolone	1.1	M
Methylprednisolone	1.5	M
6-Methylprednisolone	1.35	M
6-Methyl-F-prednisolone	1.83	M
Dexamethasone	1.0	M
Triamcinolone	1.9	M

*Elimination may be dose-dependent—e.g., the mean half-lives of phenylbutazone following intravenous doses of 10 and 50 mg/kg were 2.8 and 8.1 hours, respectively (Dayton et al., 1967).

M, metabolism; E, excretion; r, renal; b, biliary

Table 6–7 THE HALF-LIFE VALUES (IN HOURS) OF DRUGS *human*
WHICH ARE ELIMINATED MAINLY BY METABOLISM

Drug	Pony	Cow (Goat)	Pig	Dog	Cat	References	
Salicylate	1.0	0.54* (0.78)	5.9	8.6	37.6†	Davis and Westfall, 1972	*2.4 "normal dose"*
Chloramphenicol	0.9	(2.0)	1.3	4.2	5.1	Davis et al., 1972	*2.7*
Trimethoprim	3.8[b]	(0.5)[a]	2.0[a]	3.0[c]	—	a Nielsen and Rasmussen, 1972 *11.0*
						b Alexander and Collett, 1974	
						c Kaplan et al., 1970	
Sulfadimethoxine	11.3[d]	12.5**	15.5[e]	13.2*	10.2*	d Tschudi, 1972	
						e Tschudi, 1973	
Amphetamine	1.4	(0.6)	1.1	4.5	6.5	Baggot and Davis, 1973	
Quinidine	4.4	(0.85)	5.4	5.6	1.9	Neff et al., 1972	*6*

*Baggot, J. D. (1975).

**Boxenbaum, H. (1974). Research Division, Hoffmann-LaRoche Inc., Nutley, N.J.: Personal communication.

†Half-life of salicylate in the cat is dose-dependent.

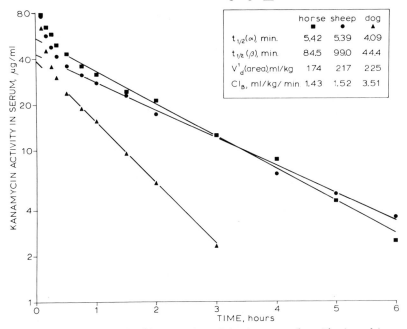

KANAMYCIN, SINGLE DOSE (10mg/kg) <u>IV</u> BOLUS

Figure 6–12 A graph of kanamycin activity in serum (logarithmic scale) as a function of time (linear scale) after intravenous dosage (10 mg/kg) of the antibiotic in dog (▲), horse (■), and sheep (•). The individual of each species for which data are plotted is representative of a group of six animals studied. Note the much steeper slope of the elimination phase (larger value of β and shorter half-life) of kanamycin disposition in the dog compared to horse and sheep (herbivorous species). Kinetic constants which describe disposition of kanamycin are given in Table 6–9.

depends upon the half-life, which also is used to predict the dosage interval of a multiple-dose regimen. The time it takes to attain the steady state level upon repetitive dosing is dependent on the half-time for elimination (half-life) of the drug.

The biological half-life of a drug may be defined using the plasma (or serum) concentration data as a point of reference, as in this book, or from the standpoint of a pharmacological effect elicited by the drug. In studying the literature one should be aware of this ambiguity and determine which criterion is used by the author(s). The values will agree only when there is a linear relationship between the drug concentration in plasma and the intensity of the observed pharmacological effect. Although there are instances in which the intensity of a pharmacological effect apparently is linearly related to the drug concentration, one cannot assume that this direct relationship exists (Levy, 1964). In such cases the time course of pharmacological effect and drug concentration are parallel (Levy and Gibaldi, 1972). It is found frequently that the intensity of a direct and reversible pharmacological effect is related linearly, over a considerable range, to the logarithm of the dose administered (Levy, 1964).

Relationships Among Dose, Elimination Rate and Duration of Pharmacological Effect

A linear relationship may be expected to exist between the duration of a pharmacological effect and the logarithm of an intravenously administered, or relatively rapidly absorbed, dose of a drug under certain conditions. These conditions include: (a) the intensity of the effect at a given time is a function of the amount of drug in the body at that time, (b) drug metabolites are inactive or very rapidly eliminated, and (c) the drug is eliminated by apparent first-order kinetics, with the elimination rate constant independent of dose (Remmer et al., 1961; Levy and Nelson, 1965; Levy, 1966; Levy and Gibaldi, 1972). This relationship may be expressed mathematically by:

$$t_d = \frac{2.3}{\beta} (\log A_0) - \frac{2.3}{\beta} (\log A_{min}) \quad \textbf{Equation 6 • 12}$$

that is,

$$t_d = \frac{2.3}{\beta} \log \left(\frac{A_0}{A_{min}} \right) \quad \textbf{Equation 6 • 13}$$

where t_d is the duration of pharmacological effect, β is the apparent first-order rate constant for drug elimination, A_0 is the intravenously injected (or very rapidly absorbed) dose, and A_{min} is the minimum effective dose (Levy and Nelson, 1965). According to Equation 6·12, a plot of duration of effect versus logarithm of dose should be linear, and the slope of the line will be equal to $2.3/\beta$. This method may be applied to determine the rate constant for drug elimination in instances in which direct measurement of drug concentration as a function of time is not possible but when the duration of a given pharmacological effect can be measured accurately (Levy, 1966). The linear relationship between duration of effect and logarithm of the dose (or amount of drug in the body) holds true only for drugs that are rapidly and homogeneously distributed and undergo exponential elimination—i.e., drugs whose disposition kinetics can be adequately described by a one-compartment open model. Implicit in this pharmacokinetic model is the assumption that a change in drug concentration in any particular tissue (e.g., at site of action) is accompanied by a corresponding change in concentration in all other tissues (including the plasma).

It can be shown for this system that the maximum intensity and duration of effect produced by a second, equal-sized dose administered immediately after disappearance of the effect of the first dose will exceed the intensity and duration of effect obtained from the initial dose (Levy, 1966). This is due to the fact that the second dose is superimposed upon the minimum effective amount of the drug that remains in the body from the first dose. Third and subsequent equal doses elicit the same intensity and duration of effect as the second dose, because when the effect subsides, the minimum effective amount remains constant. Dosage intervals chosen in relation to the duration of effect given by the second dose of drug can prevent accumulation of the drug in tissues.

Drugs which move relatively slowly in and out of distribution compartments thereby confer pharmacokinetic characteristics of a multicompartment system and elicit a considerably different time course of pharmacological effect than do drugs that are distributed in the body extremely rapidly. The qualitative nature of the relationship between duration of effect and intravenous dose for such drugs depends on whether the site of action is in the central or peripheral compartment. Unlike the single-compartment system, the duration of effect is not linearly related to the logarithm of dose (Wagner, 1968b; Gibaldi et al., 1971). Additional differences between the single- and multicompartment systems are: (a) third and subsequent equal doses administered upon recovery from the effect of preceding doses produce longer durations of effect than that of the second dose, and (b) apparently linear relationships between duration of effect and logarithm of dose can be obtained in a restricted dose range, but the slope of the line is dependent on the intensity of the effect used as the end point (Gibaldi et al., 1971). Drugs with sites of action located in relatively small and very slowly accessible compartments of a multicompartment system show a delayed onset and a prolonged duration of effect. There may be pronounced pharmacological effects at a time when no drug is detectable in the plasma. The behavior of reversibly acting drugs with so-called "hit-and-run" characteristics (e.g., the antihypertensive effect of guanethidine in humans) can be rationalized on this basis (Gibaldi et al., 1971). In general, drugs with delayed onset of effect, despite absence of significant drug accumulation in the plasma, are likely to have persistent effects and should be used with due caution.

Apparent Volume of Distribution

The apparent volume of distribution (V_d) is an important concept in the pharmacokinetic characterization of drugs. It can be defined as that volume of fluid which would be required to contain the amount of drug in the body if it were uniformly distributed at a concentration equal to that in the plasma. The assumption is made that the body behaves as a single homogeneous compartment with respect to the drug. The apparent volume of distribution does not represent an actual volume — that is, it should not be regarded as a particular physiological space within the body. The value of V_d serves as a proportionality constant relating the plasma concentration of a drug to the total amount of drug in the body at any time after distribution equilibrium has been attained:

$$C_P \cdot V_d = A_{B(t)} \qquad \textbf{Equation 6 • 14}$$

where C_P and $A_{B(t)}$ are the plasma concentration and amount of drug in the body, respectively, at time t. Caution must be exercised when selecting a method, of which there are several, for calculating the volume of distribution parameter. If a drug is truly distributed according to a one-compartment open model, the calculated value of V_d may be expected to be independent of the method used to determine it (Riegelman et al., 1968b). However, if a drug is distributed according to a multicompartment model, the value for V_d is dependent upon the kinetics (Notari, 1973).

When a two-compartment open model describes the disposition kinetics of a drug, the proportionality constant, $V_{d(\beta)}$, which relates drug concentration in the plasma to the total amount of drug in the body at any time after attainment of pseudodistribution equilibrium may be obtained from:

$$V_{d(\beta)} = \frac{k_{el} \cdot V_c}{\beta} = \frac{V_c}{f_c} \qquad \textbf{Equation 6 • 15}$$

where k_{el} is the specific elimination rate constant for loss of drug from the central compartment; and β is the overall rate constant for elimination of drug from the body; V_c is the volume of the central compartment; and f_c is the fraction of the amount of drug in the body that is contained in the central compartment. The "area" method provides another satisfactory way of calculating the volume of distribution parameter:

$$V_{d(area)} = \frac{Dose}{(Area) \cdot \beta} = \frac{Dose}{(A/\alpha + B/\beta) \cdot \beta}$$

Equation 6 • 16

where (Area) is the total area under the plasma drug concentration versus time curve, plotted on arithmetic coordinates, from $t = 0$ to $t = \infty$, and is expressed in units of mg-min/liter. The area method provides a volume of distribution, $V_{d(area)}$, which is absolutely equivalent to the volume of distribution at pseudodistribution equilibrium, $V_{d(\beta)}$, as rigorously defined in the two-compartment open model (Gibaldi et al., 1969):

$$V_{d(\beta)} = \frac{V_c}{f_c} = V_{d(area)} \qquad \text{Equation 6 • 17}$$

After single intravenous doses the apparent volume of distribution may sometimes be calculated by the "extrapolation" method (Nelson, 1961):

$$V_{d(B)} = \frac{Dose}{B} \qquad \text{Equation 6 • 18}$$

where B (in units of concentration) is the zero-time intercept of the terminal exponential (β) phase of drug decline in plasma after intravenous administration of a single dose. Since the extrapolation method neglects the distributive or α phase of drug disposition, it should be used to calculate V_d only for drugs (given as single doses intravenously) whose disposition kinetics can be described adequately by a one-compartment open model. If data are best represented by the two-compartment open model, the volume of distribution calculated by the extrapolation method (which really assumes that the one-compartment open model applies) will be larger than the value obtained by the area method and, consequently, will overestimate the magnitude of this parameter. Values of V_d for some antimicrobial agents calculated by the different methods are compared (Table 6–8).

Table 6–8   THE APPARENT SPECIFIC VOLUMES OF DISTRIBUTION
(ml/kg) OF ANTIMICROBIAL AGENTS IN DOGS (A SINGLE
INTRAVENOUS DOSE (mg/kg) OF EACH DRUG
WAS ADMINISTERED)

Drug	$V'_{d(B)} = \text{Dose}/B$	$V'_{d(\beta)} =$ $(k_{el} \cdot V_c)/\beta$	$V'_{d(area)} =$ $\text{Dose}/(\text{Area})\beta$	$V'_{d(ss)} =$ $\left(\dfrac{k_{12} + k_{21}}{k_{21}}\right) V'_c$
Penicillin G	273	156	156	115
Kanamycin	278	255	255	236
Gentamicin	448	335	335	260
Sulfadimethoxine	523	410	410	342
Oxytetracycline	3100	2096	2096	1508*

*Three-compartment open model:

$$V'_{d(ss)} = \left(\frac{k_{21}k_{31} + k_{12}k_{31} + k_{21}k_{13}}{k_{21} \cdot k_{31}}\right) V'_c$$

The apparent volume of distribution of a drug gives an idea of the extent or magnitude of its distribution, but provides no clue as to whether distribution of the drug is uniform or restricted to certain tissues. A large apparent volume of distribution implies wide distribution or extensive tissue binding, or both. Lipid-soluble organic bases (e.g., amphetamine, morphine, quinidine, lidocaine, diazepam) are widely distributed in body fluids and tissues, and have large volumes of distribution which exceed the actual volume of the body (>1 liter/kg). The low lipid-solubility of aminoglycoside antibiotics restricts the distribution of these organic bases ($V'_d < 0.3$ liter/kg). Although aminoglycosides have a small magnitude of distribution, they are avidly bound to renal tissue, a fact which could never be deduced from the volume of distribution parameter. The volume of distribution of a drug may be numerically the same as the extracellular fluid volume of the body, but this coincidence should not be interpreted as meaning that the drug is uniformly distributed in extracellular fluid or even limited to this physiological compartment. Organic acids that are predominantly ionized in plasma (e.g., salicylates, phenylbutazone, penicillins) have small volumes of distribution (<0.25 liter/kg). The sulfonamides and pentobarbitone are weak organic acids which exist as both the nonionized and the ionized forms in plasma, penetrate biological membranes with relative ease, and have volumes of distribution that may be considered intermediate (0.3 to 0.8 liter/kg). Volume of distribution, which is a proportionality constant and not a physiological volume, is a most useful pharmacokinetic term; it is essential for computing the dose that must be administered to produce a desired plasma drug concentration. The apparent volume of distribution of a drug is the sum of the volumes of the central and peripheral distribution compartments for the drug.

The average amount of drug in the body at steady state ($\overline{A}_B^\infty$) upon repetitive dosing in a two-compartment open system is related to the average steady state plasma level ($\overline{C}_P^\infty$) by the apparent volume of distribution at steady state, $V_{d(ss)}$, even though the average plasma level is dependent on $V_{d(\beta)}$ (Perrier and Gibaldi, 1973):

$$\overline{A}_B^\infty = \overline{C}_P^\infty \cdot V_{d(ss)}^\infty \qquad \text{Equation 6 • 19}$$

Multiplication of $\overline{C}_P^\infty$ by $V_{d(\beta)}$, the apparent volume of distribution at pseudodistribution equilibrium, results in an overestimation of the average amount of drug in the body at steady state, the magnitude of which depends on the relative distribution and elimination parameters of the drug. The volume of distribution at the steady state can be calculated for a drug (given by repetitive dosing) that confers upon the body the characteristics of a two-compartment model:

$$V_{d(ss)} = \left(\frac{k_{12} + k_{21}}{k_{21}}\right) V_c \qquad \text{Equation 6 • 20}$$

where k_{12} and k_{21} are the first-order rate constants for distribution between central and peripheral compartments, and V_c is the volume of the central compartment (Riegelman et al., 1968b). This method assumes that the rate of change in the amount of drug in the peripheral compartment is zero; this situation occurs at only one instant following the intravenous injection of a single dose. The necessary condition of no net drug transfer between compartments holds only at that single point in time when the drug concentration in the peripheral compartment has reached a maximum. $V_{d(ss)}$ is useful mainly when a steady state plasma (or serum) concentration of drug is reached during constant intravenous infusion. In this situation, $V_{d(ss)}$ is related to the plasma concentration of drug and the amount of drug in the body at infusion equilibrium (C_P^{ss} and A_B^{ss}, respectively) by the equation (Gibaldi, 1969):

$$V_{d(ss)} = \frac{A_B^{ss}}{C_P^{ss}} \qquad \text{Equation 6 • 21}$$

where $$A_B^{ss} = \text{Dose}\left(1 - \frac{\int_0^T C_P\, dt}{\int_0^\infty C_P\, dt}\right) \qquad \text{Equation 6 • 22}$$

The integrals $\int_0^T C_P \, dt$ and $\int_0^\infty C_P \, dt$ are the respective areas under the plasma concentration versus time curves from time zero (initiation) to T and time zero to infinity upon constant intravenous infusion, where T is the time at which infusion is terminated (Perrier and Gibaldi, 1973). Assuming that elimination occurs only from the central compartment, $V_{d(ss)}$ can be determined regardless of the number of distribution compartments in the pharmacokinetic model and can be employed to estimate the amount of drug in the body at infusion equilibrium and during steady state upon repetitive dosing.

Drug Levels in the Central and Peripheral (Tissue) Compartments

Following rapid intravenous injection of a drug that distributes in the body according to a two-compartment open model with elimination occurring from the central compartment, the time course of the amount of drug in the compartments can be described by equations $6 \cdot 23$ and $6 \cdot 24$.

For the central compartment:

$$A_c = \frac{A_0(\alpha - k_{21})}{\alpha - \beta} e^{-\alpha t} + \frac{A_0(k_{21} - \beta)}{\alpha - \beta} e^{-\beta t} \qquad \textbf{Equation 6 • 23}$$

For the tissue compartment:

$$A_T = \frac{k_{12} A_0}{\beta - \alpha} e^{-\alpha t} + \frac{k_{12} A_0}{\alpha - \beta} e^{-\beta t} \qquad \textbf{Equation 6 • 24}$$

where A_0 is the amount of drug in the central compartment at time zero and is equal to the intravenous dose, and A_c and A_T are the amounts of drug in the central and peripheral (tissue) compartments, respectively, at any time t. After distribution equilibrium has been reached, the plasma and peripheral compartment levels decline in parallel, since the slope of the terminal exponential (postdistributive) phase is $-\beta/2.303$.

An analogue computer can be used to simulate the curves describing the level of drug (expressed as fraction of the single intravenous dose) in the central and peripheral compartments as a function of time, as well as the fraction of drug eliminated. For any drug whose disposition kinetics can be described by a two-compartment open model the simulated drug level curves are related to the calculated value of C_P^0 (initial plasma drug concentration immediately following rapid intravenous injection, $A + B$) and are based on the individual rate constants (k_{12}, k_{21}, k_{el}) associated with the model. The simulated serum and tissue level curves for erythromycin and tylosin in cows, ketamine in a cat and penicillin G in a dog are shown in Figures 6–13 to 6–16. A considerable amount of information on disposition of a drug in a particular species can be deduced by inspection and study of the drug level curves. Each figure is based on data obtained in a single animal, which was considered representative of the group of animals (in most cases six individuals) used in the drug disposition study. A single dose of drug was administered as an intravenous bolus, and blood samples for assay of drug content were collected at precisely timed intervals. Consider the disposition of erythromycin and tylosin, which are macrolide antibiotics, separately and compare the levels produced by the same dose (12.5 mg/kg) given intravenously to normal cows. The close correlation between the experimental, time-dependent plasma level (serum level in the case of antibiotics) data and the computer-simulated curve for the central compartment indicates that the two-compartment open model adequately describes the time course of plasma drug levels. The tissue level of erythromycin reached a peak of 43 per cent of the intravenous dose at 67 min. At 6 hours, the percentages of the dose of erythromycin in the central and tissue compartments were 6 and 19

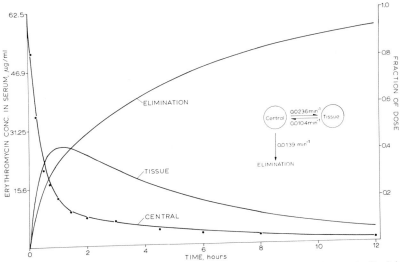

Figure 6–13 Relationship of measured erythromycin activity (concentration) in serum (•) as a function of time to computer-simulated curves showing the fraction of the administered dose in the central and peripheral (or tissue) compartments, as well as that eliminated during the same time period. The curves are based on values of the individual first-order rate constants associated with the two-compartment open model (inset), which describes disposition kinetics of the drug (see Fig. 6–4 and Table 6–1). (From Baggot, J. D., and Gingerich, D. A. [1976]: *Res. vet. Sci.,* 21:318–323.)

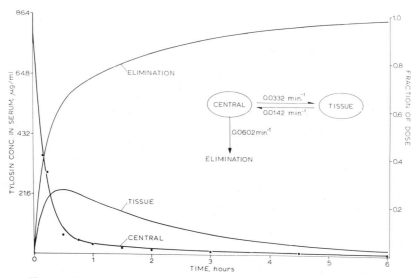

Figure 6–14 Simulated curves of tylosin levels (as fraction of dose) in the central and tissue compartments and the fraction eliminated as a function of time. A single intravenous dose (12.5 mg/kg) was given to a cow and decline of tylosin activity in serum (•) was measured. A scheme of the two-compartment open model and calculated values of the microconstants are shown. (From Baggot, J. D., and Gingerich, D. A. [1976]: *Res. vet. Sci.*, 21:318–323.)

per cent, respectively, with 75 per cent of the dose having been eliminated. The ratio of drug level in the tissue compartment to central compartment at the time pseudodistribution equilibrium was reached was 2.27 (obtained from drug level curves at 67 min), which is equal to the calculated value of k_{12}/k_{21}. This is the only instant at which the rate of change in amount of drug in the peripheral compartment is zero, and the apparent volume of distribution at steady state, $V_{d(ss)}$, provides a good estimate of V_d when a drug is given as a single dose. The peak level of tylosin in the tissue compartment (26.5 per cent of the dose) was present at 30 min. Tylosin levels in the central and tissue compartments at 4 hours after intravenous administration of a single dose (12.5 mg/kg) were 1 and 5 per cent of the dose, respectively, and 94 per cent had been eliminated at that time. At the instant apparent distribution equilibrium was attained, the ratio of drug level in central compartment to peripheral compartment was 2.34 (k_{12}/k_{21}). The half-life of each antibiotic was calculated from the slope of the least squares linear regression line which represents the terminal exponential phase of the decline in serum drug activity (concentration). The half-life (mean ± S.D., $n = 6$) of erythromycin was 3.16 ± 0.44

hours, while that of tylosin was 1.62 ± 0.17 hours (Baggot and Gingerich, 1976). The apparent specific volumes of distribution, $V^1_{d(area)}$, were 0.79 ± 0.17 liter/kg and 1.10 ± 0.45 liter/kg for erythromycin and tylosin, respectively. The large apparent volume of distribution implies wide extravascular distribution and/or tissue binding, and supports the wide overall tissue-to-plasma level ratio which exists at all times after pseudodistribution equilibrium is attained. By inspecting the tissue and plasma level curves for either antibiotic one can see that the overall tissue-to-plasma level ratio did not remain constant and was equal to the calculated value (k_{12}/k_{21}) only at the single time at which pseudodistribution equilibrium (peak of tissue level curve) was reached. This discrepancy may be explained by the fact that distribution equilibrium was never fully attained.

Ketamine, a dissociative anesthetic agent, is eliminated from the body by hepatic biotransformation and excretion processes. When the drug was given as a single intravenous dose (25 mg/kg) to cats, the plasma concentration–time profile consisted of a rapid distribution phase $(t_{1/2\,(\alpha)} = 3$ min) and much slower elimination (β) phase. The half-life (mean $\pm$ S.D., $n=6$) of ketamine was 66.9 ± 24.1 min, and was

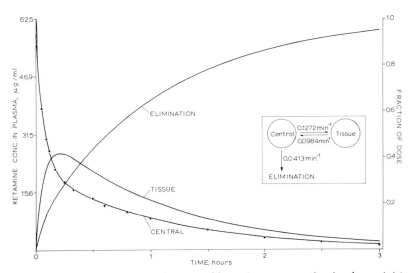

Figure 6–15 Relationship of measured ketamine concentration in plasma (•) to computer-simulated curves of ketamine levels (as fraction of dose) in the central and tissue compartments as a function of time. A curve showing the fraction of dose eliminated is also given. The data were obtained after intravenous administration of a dose (25 mg/kg) of ketamine hydrochloride to a cat (see Figure 6–6); values of the constants which describe disposition kinetics of the drug are given in Table 6–1. A scheme of the two-compartment open model showing values of first-order rate constants associated with the model is given in inset. (From Baggot, J. D., and Blake, J. W. [1976]: *Arch. int. Pharmacodyn. Thér.*, 220:115–124.)

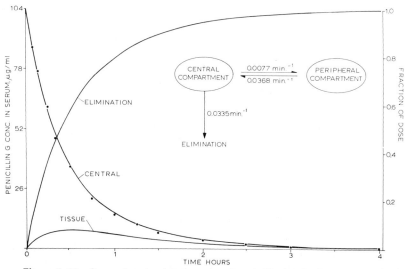

Figure 6–16   Computer-simulated curves of penicillin levels (fraction of dose) in the central and tissue compartments. The decline of penicillin activity in serum (•) after giving a single intravenous dose (10 mg/kg) of potassium penicillin G to a dog is shown (arithmetic coordinates). Compare the relative positions on the graph of the serum and tissue level curves with the curves shown in the three previous figures. The elimination curve represents the cumulative amount (in terms of fraction of dose) of penicillin excreted in the urine.

independent of the route of parenteral administration. A large apparent specific volume of distribution, $V'_{d(B)} = 1.714 \pm 0.743$ liter/kg, was obtained (Baggot and Blake, 1976). Disposition of ketamine was described by a two-compartment open model. The simulated curves of drug level in the central and tissue compartments as a function of time and the fraction of the dose eliminated show that at 90 min after injecting the drug 8.6 per cent of the dose was present in the central compartment, 13.4 per cent was distributed in tissues and 78 per cent of the dose had been eliminated (Fig. 6–15). The tissue level is the amount of drug contained in the tissues or peripheral compartment and may not reflect the drug concentration at the site of action, even though the site of action is located in the peripheral compartment. The peak tissue level (42 per cent of the dose) was present between 11 and 14 min, at which time the overall tissue-to-plasma level ratio was 1.3:1. The tissue level exceeded the level of drug in the plasma from 8.5 min after giving the intravenous dose.

The tissue level curve for penicillin G, an organic acid (pK_a 2.7), contrasts with that of ketamine, a lipophilic organic base. Ionization and low degree of lipid-solubility limit distribution of penicillin G by restricting tissue penetration of the antibiotic, which is reflected by the small apparent volume of distribution (<0.2 liter/kg) and low overall tissue level (Fig. 6–16). At 30 min after giving a single intravenous dose (10 mg/kg) of potassium penicillin G to a dog, the overall tissue-to-serum level of the drug was 1:5. At 3 hours, a similar but very small percentage (0.75 per cent) of the dose was present in both the central and tissue compartments. Since the antibiotic is eliminated entirely by renal mechanisms (glomerular filtration and carrier-mediated tubular excretion), the elimination curve corresponds to penicillin levels in the urine. When a time period of six half-lives of the drug had elapsed (6 × 31.5 min) the cumulative amount excreted accounts for 98.4 per cent of the dose.

Kanamycin, a polar organic base, was given by intravenous injection at the same dosage rate (10 mg/kg) to normal dogs, sheep and horses. The decline in serum kanamycin activity in an individual animal representative of each species is shown in Figure 6–12. After pseudo-distribution equilibrium was attained, the serum levels of kanamycin were lower in dogs than in sheep and horses. This was due mainly to elimination (excretion) of a greater fraction of the dose during the initial phase (first 30 min after I.V. dosage) in dogs (45 per cent) compared with sheep (24 per cent) and horses (25 per cent). The half-life (mean ± S.D., $n = 6$) of kanamycin was significantly shorter in dogs (0.97 ± 0.31 hours) than in sheep (1.74 ± 0.23 hours) and horses (1.45 ± 0.15 hours). The polarity of this compound restricts tissue penetration, which is reflected by the small apparent volume of distribution,

Table 6–9 PHARMACOKINETIC PARAMETERS WHICH DESCRIBE DISPOSITION OF KANAMYCIN AFTER INTRAVENOUS INJECTION OF A SINGLE DOSE (10 mg/kg)

Kinetic Parameter	Units	Dog	Sheep	Horse
C_P^0	μg/ml	103.8	108.8	109.0
A	μg/ml	65.4	66.4	55.0
α	min^{-1}	0.1693	0.1286	0.1279
$t_{1/2(\alpha)}$	min	4.09	5.39	5.42
B	μg/ml	38.4	42.4	54.0
β	min^{-1}	0.0156	0.0070	0.0082
$t_{1/2(\beta)}$	min	44.4	99.0	84.5
k_{12}	min^{-1}	0.0760	0.0647	0.0531
k_{21}	min^{-1}	0.0725	0.0544	0.0675
k_{el}	min^{-1}	0.0364	0.0165	0.0155
V'_c	ml/kg	96	92	92
$V'_{d(area)}$	ml/kg	225	217	174
Cl_B	ml/kg/min	3.51	1.52	1.43
k_{12}/k_{21}		1.05	1.19	0.79
Body weight	kg	11.4	36.4	477.3

typical of aminoglycoside antibiotics but unusual for an organic base. The two-compartment open model was used to describe the disposition kinetics of the drug (Table 6–9). Since elimination is almost entirely by renal excretion (glomerular filtration) the simulated elimination curve, generated by an analogue computer and based on individual rate constants associated with the two-compartment open model, represents the cumulative amount of kanamycin excreted in urine. The kanamycin levels (expressed as fraction of the dose) in the serum and tissue compartments and in the urine as a function of time are presented in Figures 6–17, 6–18 and 6–19. The close fit of the data points to the simulated serum level curves shows that the two-compartment model adequately describes disposition of this drug. The peak tissue level (35 per cent of the dose) was present between 19 and 24 min in dogs, and the overall tissue levels were somewhat higher than serum

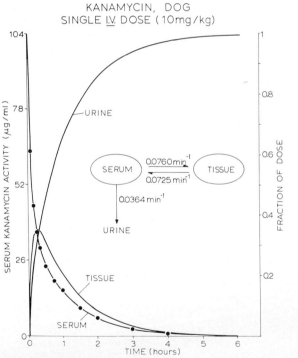

Figure 6–17 Disposition of kanamycin in the dog after intravenous dosage. Analogue computer-generated curves of kanamycin levels (as fraction of dose administered) in the serum and tissue compartments and the cumulative amount excreted in the urine as a function of time are shown. Closed circles (•) represent the activity of kanamycin in serum. A graph of the decline in serum kanamycin activity, plotted on semilogarithmic paper, is given in Figure 6–12.

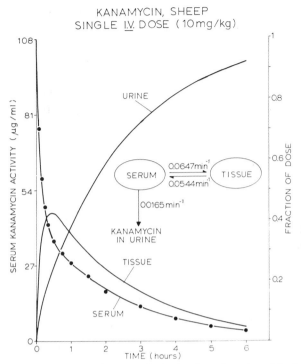

Figure 6-18 Disposition of kanamycin in the sheep based on data derived from decline of the antibiotic activity in serum after intravenous administration of a single dose. Closed circles (•) represent the activity of kanamycin in serum. A graph of the decline in serum kanamycin activity, plotted on semilogarithmic paper, is given in Figure 6-12.

levels after pseudodistribution equilibrium was reached. However, comparison of serum and tissue level curves shows that serum kanamycin activity could be used to predict amount of drug in the body ($C_P \cdot V_d$) and tissue level at any time after attainment of pseudodistribution equilibrium. The urine level (amount of drug) is approximately equal to dose minus twice serum level. Although the same generalities can be applied to kanamycin levels in the tissue compartment and urine of the three species, there are interesting differences between antibiotic levels in tissue compartments of the sheep and horse, even though their serum level curves are closely similar. While the peak tissue level was present at the same time (25 min) in both species, a greater fraction of the dose (42 per cent compared with 34 per cent) was distributed in the tissue compartment of sheep. This difference is reflected in the relative values of the k_{12}/k_{21} ratio. In each animal

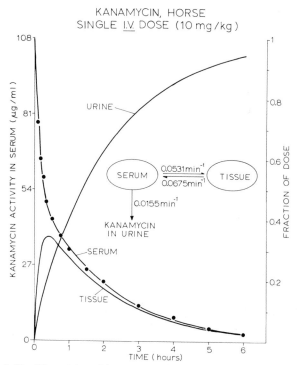

Figure 6–19 Disposition of kanamycin in the horse based on data derived from decline of the antibiotic activity in serum after intravenous administration of a single dose. Closed circles (•) represent the activity of kanamycin in serum. A graph of the decline in serum kanamycin activity, plotted on semilogarithmic paper, is given in Figure 6–12.

species, the serum and tissue level curves for kanamycin declined in an approximately parallel fashion. At 6 hours, which is approximately four half-lives of the drug in the herbivorous species, 92 per cent and 94 per cent of the intravenous dose were eliminated in sheep and horses, respectively. Owing to the shorter half-life of kanamycin in dogs, an equivalent amount of the drug was eliminated in a 3 hour period. The overall tissue level–time curve would not reflect selective binding of a small fraction of the dose to a particular tissue. This inadequacy limits usefulness of the analogue computer-generated curves in drug residue studies, in that various organs and tissues of the body must eventually be analyzed for drug content. The greatest value of the simulated drug level curves in residue studies is in predicting the time after dosing animals at which tissue samples should be obtained and analyzed for drug content.

Body Clearance

Clearance of a drug, which is defined as the volume of blood cleared of the drug by the various elimination processes (biotransformation and excretion) per unit time, is a pharmacokinetic concept of considerable importance. The (total) body clearance is the product of the apparent volume of distribution and the overall elimination rate constant:

$$Cl_B = k_{el} \cdot V_c$$

$$= \beta \cdot V_{d(\text{area})} = \left(\frac{0.693}{t_{1/2}}\right) V_{d(\text{area})}$$

Equation 6 • 25

The area method for estimating the apparent volume of distribution is applicable following parenteral and oral administration of a drug, provided the dose is completely absorbed. The body clearance may be estimated by dividing the dose administered by the total area under the plasma drug level versus time curve. The area under the curve (AUC) may be calculated according to:

$$\text{AUC} = \int_0^{t*} C_P dt + \frac{C_P(t*)}{\beta}$$

Equation 6 • 26

where $t*$ is the time at which the last blood sample was collected, $C_P(t*)$ is the last measured concentration of the drug in plasma and β is the overall elimination rate constant. The area from time zero to $t*$ can be estimated using the trapezoidal rule. For most drugs the half-life is a complex function encompassing several discrete pharmacological processes: drug distribution, biotransformation and renal excretion. Clearance, on the other hand, permits expression of the rates of drug removal from the body in a way that is independent of these processes (Rowland et al., 1973). The half-life and body clearance values of various antimicrobial agents (each given as a single intravenous dose) in dogs are tabulated in order of increasing half-life (Table 6–10). The data show that a short half-life should not be equated with a high clearance, since the clearance parameter comprises a volume as well as a rate component. Unlike β and $t_{1/2}$, which are hybrid parameters and depend upon k_{12}, k_{21} and k_{el}, body clearance changes exactly in proportion to k_{el} (Jusko and Gibaldi, 1972). V_c is mathematically independent of k_{el}.

Table 6-10   CLEARANCE OF ANTIMICROBIAL AGENTS IN DOGS

Drug	Process(es) of Elimination	$t_{1/2}$ (min)	$V'_{d(area)}$ (ml/kg)	Cl_B (ml/kg/min)
Penicillin G	E (r)	30	156	3.6
Ampicillin	E (r)	48	270	3.9
Tylosin	E (b + r) + M	54	1700	21.82
Kanamycin	E (r)	58	255	3.05
Gentamicin	E (r)	75	335	3.10
Trimethoprim	M + E (r)	180*	1700	6.55
Chloramphenicol	M	252	1770	4.87
Sulfisoxazole	E (r) + M	270*	300	0.77
Oxytetracycline	E (r)	360	2096	4.03
Sulfadimethoxine	E(r) + M	792*	410	0.36
Compounds used to estimate renal function				
[125]I-Iothalamate	Glomerular filtration	31.5	245	5.4
[131]I-Iodohippurate	Glomerular filtration + Tubular secretion	15.8	350	15.3

*$t_{1/2}$ is dependent on urinary pH.
M = metabolism; E = excretion; r = renal; b = biliary.

In the acute stage of systemic infections, when the febrile reaction is present, tissue penetration of some antimicrobial agents may be increased (reflected by an increased magnitude of the apparent volume of distribution parameter) and their half-lives increased (due to a smaller fraction of the dose being present in the central compartment and available for elimination), so that no change is seen in their clearance values. This situation was found to exist for penicillin G when the disposition kinetics of the drug were compared in normal beagles and in beagles during the acute stage, based on febrile response, of an induced generalized streptococcal infection (Table 6-11). Intravenous therapy with penicillin G was initiated 48 hours after giving the challenging dose (3×10^8 colony forming units) of a group C beta hemolytic streptococcus (*Streptococcus zooepidemicus*) by intravenous injection. The dosage regimen consisted of a series of single intravenous doses (10 mg/kg) of potassium penicillin G, which were administered at 12 hour intervals. It is interesting to note that values of the kinetic parameters during the seventh dosage interval, after acute stage of infection had subsided, were returning to normal. The shifts in relative amounts of penicillin G in serum and tissue compartments are clearly shown in the simulated curves, which were generated by means of an analogue computer programmed with individual rate

Table 6–11 DISPOSITION KINETICS OF PENICILLIN G IN NORMAL
AND INFECTED (INDUCED STREPTOCOCCAL INFECTION)
BEAGLES FOLLOWING INTRAVENOUS DOSAGE (10 mg/kg) WITH
POTASSIUM PENICILLIN G, GIVEN AS SINGLE DOSE TO NORMAL
BEAGLES AND AS SERIES OF SINGLE DOSES (12 HOUR INTERVAL
BETWEEN SUCCESSIVE DOSES) TO INFECTED BEAGLES

Kinetic Parameter	Units	Normal ($n = 8$) Single Dose Mean $\pm$ S.D.	Infected ($n = 4$) First Dosage Interval Mean $\pm$ S.D.	Infected ($n = 4$) Seventh Dosage Interval Mean $\pm$ S.D.
A	μg/ml	72.0 ± 24.4	75.5 ± 14.5	84.0 ± 37.5
B	μg/ml	36.6 ± 9.0	36.8 ± 19.6	41.4 ± 14.3
$t_{1/2(\alpha)}$	min	11.9 ± 2.6	8.5 ± 2.3	8.9 ± 2.5
$t_{1/2(\beta)}$	min	30.0 ± 3.5	40.0 ± 5.6	35.2 ± 4.4
k_{12}	min^{-1}	0.008 ± 0.004	0.029 ± 0.016	0.022 ± 0.016
k_{21}	min^{-1}	0.036 ± 0.008	0.040 ± 0.012	0.042 ± 0.010
k_{el}	min^{-1}	0.040 ± 0.008	0.042 ± 0.012	0.040 ± 0.008
V'_c	ml/kg	94.8 ± 18	91.1 ± 14.9	89.5 ± 38.5
V'_d	ml/kg	156 ± 13	214 ± 77	168 ± 42.6
Cl_B	ml/kg/min	3.64 ± 0.39	3.70 ± 1.26	3.40 ± 1.20
$C_{P(4\ hr)}$	μg/ml	0.24 ± 0.13	0.58 ± 0.29	0.27 ± 0.18

constants associated with the two-compartment open model. The
microconstants for penicillin G distribution and elimination were
calculated for each animal, and mean values for normal dogs and for
infected dogs during the first and seventh dosage intervals were then
computed. No data points are associated with the simulated mean
serum level curves. In normal dogs given a single intravenous dose
(10 mg/kg) of potassium penicillin G, the tissue level maximum (7 per
cent of the dose) was present from 25 to 35 minutes after drug administration, during which time the serum level declined from 33 per cent
to 24 per cent of the dose (Fig. 6–20). The overall tissue-to-serum
level ratio at 30 min was 0.25:1, which was close to the value of
k_{12}/k_{21} ($= 0.23$). During the acute febrile stage of the streptococcal
infection, penetration of penicillin G into the tissues was greatly enhanced. A far greater amount of the antibiotic was present in the
tissue compartment throughout the time course of the drug in the body.
A maximum tissue level of 21 per cent of the dose was present between
20 and 28 min after administration of the first dose of penicillin G
(Fig. 6–21). At 24 min, the overall tissue-to-serum level ratio was
0.78:1. The tissue level of the antibiotic exceeded the serum level
from 33 min, unlike the situation in normal dogs, in which serum level
was higher than tissue level throughout six half-lives of the drug.
After administration of the seventh dose of potassium penicillin G to

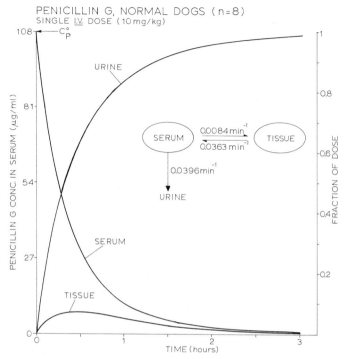

Figure 6-20 Simulated curves of penicillin levels (fraction of dose) in the serum and tissue compartments as a function of time. The urine level curve represents cumulative amount of penicillin excreted in the urine. Curves are based on data derived from the decline of penicillin activity in serum after intravenous administration of a single dose (10 mg/kg) of potassium penicillin G to normal dogs. The curves were generated by an analogue computer, which was programmed with individual first-order rate constants associated with the two-compartment open model (inset).

infected dogs, the maximum tissue level (17 per cent of the dose) was present between 22 and 28 min (Fig. 6–22). At 25 min, the overall tissue-to-serum level ratio for penicillin G was 0.56:1, in good agreement with k_{12}/k_{21} (0.53). The seventh dosage interval is a subacute stage of the infection, the febrile response having subsided. The simulated curves show serum and tissue levels to be the same from 1.25 hours after administering the seventh dose of drug. The disposition kinetics of the antibiotic appear to be returning toward the values found in the normal dogs. Since the serum level curves are almost the same in normal and infected animals (at 1 hour, for example, 11 to 12 per cent of the dose is present in the central compartment), the increased tissue levels in the infected animals occur at the expense of urinary drug levels, which are decreased. Induced fever in both dogs and humans resulted in correspondingly lower concentrations of gentamicin in serum than when the same subject was afebrile. In humans particularly, other parameters of gentamicin disposition, such as (serum) half-life and amount excreted in urine during a 6 hour period after drug administration, were not significantly altered by fever (Pennington et al., 1975).

Body clearance, which is a measure of the functional ability of a substance to be removed by the organs of elimination, is the sum of all clearance processes in the body. Renal clearance is that fraction of the body clearance attributable to excretion of unchanged drug by the kidneys. When a drug is excreted partly or entirely unchanged in the urine, its renal clearance (ml/min) can be estimated by dividing the rate of urinary excretion of the drug (mg/min) by the plasma concentra-

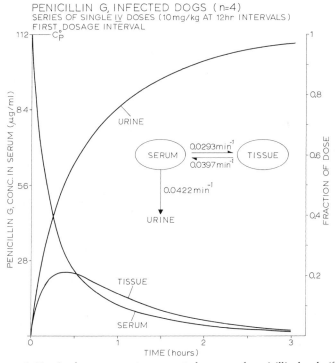

Figure 6–21 Analogue computer-generated curves of penicillin levels (fraction of dose) in the serum and tissue compartments and in the urine of dogs during the acute febrile stage of an induced streptococcal infection. Curves are based on data derived from the decline of penicillin activity in serum of infected dogs given the first of a series (12 hour dosage interval) of single doses (10 mg/kg) of potassium penicillin G by intravenous injection. The drug confers two-compartment model characteristics on the body.

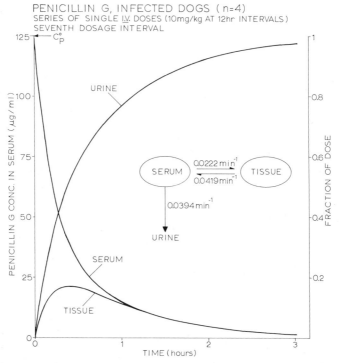

Figure 6–22 Analogue computer-generated curves of penicillin levels (fraction of dose) in the serum and tissue compartments and in the urine of dogs during the subacute (recovery) stage of an induced streptococcal infection. Curves are based on data derived from the decline of serum penicillin activity after intravenous adminis-tration of the seventh dose (10 mg/kg) of a series of penicillin doses given at 12 hour intervals to infected dogs. Compare the curves in Figures 6–20, 6–21 and 6–22 and note the intermediate position of the tissue level versus time curve relating to subacute stage of infection. It appears that extent of drug distribution (degree of tissue pene-tration) is returning to normal level after being greatly increased during febrile state.

tion (mg/ml) at the midpoint of the urine collection period. Alter-natively, one can estimate renal clearance by multiplying the body clearance value by that fraction of the administered dose (assuming complete absorption) that is excreted unchanged in the urine. Body clearance of penicillins and aminoglycosides is essentially renal clear-ance, since these antibiotics are excreted unchanged in the urine. Pentobarbitone is eliminated entirely by hepatic biotransformation, so that body clearance of this drug represents metabolic clearance. The clearance values (ml/kg/min) for pentobarbitone in dogs, horses and sheep are 1.49, 6.16 and 8.40, respectively.

   The usefulness of (biologic) half-life and body clearance as indices of hepatic elimination for drugs that are metabolized in the liver is highly dependent upon the pharmacokinetics of the particular drug under consideration (Gibaldi and Perrier, 1975). For drugs that confer multicompartment characteristics on the body, biologic half-life is a function not only of elimination but also of distribution. Hence, its value as an index of hepatic elimination becomes very questionable. Clearance, on the other hand, is a direct measure of hepatic elimination regardless of the number of compartments a drug becomes distributed into in the body, provided that there is minimal first-pass effect on oral administration. Following the intravenous administration of drugs subject to significant first-pass metabolism, when rate of hepatic biotransformation exceeds transfer of drug from plasma to site of biotransformation (hepatic blood flow), one would not anticipate a demonstrable change in the half-life or body clearance values even though substantial changes occur in hepatic clearance. After oral drug administration, however, where the drug must pass through the liver prior to reaching the systemic circulation, changes in hepatic clearance are reflected quantitatively by changes in the area under the plasma concentration versus time curve (Gibaldi and Perrier, 1975).

The clearance of certain substances can be used as an index of renal function (inulin, ^{125}I-iothalamate:GFR; para-aminohippurate, ^{131}I-iodohippurate:ERPF) or hepatic function (Bromsulphalein or BSP). Great care must be exercised in the interpretation of clearance values obtained, since factors other than abnormal function of the organ being assessed may influence clearance of the test substance. If a carrier- or enzyme-mediated process is involved in elimination of the test substance, inhibition of the elimination process caused by another agent (drug interaction) will decrease the clearance value obtained. Fever, even a mild febrile response, may alter disposition of the agent used to measure function of an eliminating organ. It has been shown in humans that mild to moderate febrile reactions lead to significant alterations in BSP excretion, by producing increased reflux from the liver to the plasma and decreased relative hepatic storage capacity (Blaschke et al., 1973).

REFERENCES

Alexander, F., and Collett, R. A. (1974): Some observations on the pharmacokinetics of trimethoprim in the horse. *Brit. J. Pharmac.*, *52*:142.

Arnold, K., and Gerber, N. (1970): The rate of decline of diphenylhydantoin in human plasma. *Clin. Pharmac. Ther.*, *11*:121–134.

Baggot, J. D., and Blake, J. W. (1976): Disposition kinetics of ketamine in the domestic cat. *Arch. Int. Pharmacodyn. Ther.*, *220*:115–124.

Baggot, J. D., and Davis, L. E. (1973): A comparative study of the pharmacokinetics of amphetamine. *Res. Vet. Sci.*, *14*:207–215.

Baggot, J. D., and Gingerich, D. A. (1976): Pharmacokinetic interpretation of erythro-

188   PRINCIPLES OF PHARMACOKINETICS

mycin and tylosin activity in serum after intravenous administration of a single dose to cows. *Res. vet. Sci., 21*:318–323.

Berlin, C. M., Stackman, J. M., and Vesell, E. S. (1975): Quinine-induced alterations in drug disposition. *Clin. Pharmacol. Ther., 18*:670–679.

Blaschke, T. F., Elin, R. J., Berk, P. D., Song, C. S., and Wolff, S. M. (1973): Effect of induced fever on sulfobromophthalein kinetics in man. *Ann. intern. Med., 78*:221–226.

Boxenbaum, H. G., and Kaplan, S. A. (1975): Potential source of error in absorption rate calculations. *J. pharmacokinet. Biopharm., 3*:257–264.

Bridges, J. W., Kibby, M. R., Walker, S. R., and Williams, R. T. (1968): Species differences in the metabolism of sulfadimethoxine. *Biochem. J., 109*:851–856.

Burns, J. J., Rose, R. K., Chenkin, T., Goldman, A., Schulert, A., and Brodie, B. B. (1953): The physiological disposition of phenylbutazone (Butazolidin) in man, and a method for its estimation in biological material. *J. Pharmacol. exp. Ther., 109*:346–357.

Burns, J. J., Yu, T. F., Dayton, P. G., Gutman, A. B., and Brodie, B. B. (1960): Biochemical pharmacological considerations of phenylbutazone and its analogues. *Ann. N.Y. Acad. Sci., 86*:253–262.

Byron, P. R., and Notari, R. E. (1976): Critical analysis of "flip-flop" phenomenon in two-compartment pharmacokinetic model. *J. pharm. Sci., 65*:1140–1144.

Davis, L. E., Neff, C. A., Baggot, J. D., and Powers, T. E. (1972): Pharmacokinetics of chloramphenicol in domesticated animals. *Am. J. vet. Res., 33*:2259–2266.

Davis, L. E., and Westfall, B. A. (1972): Species differences in biotransformation and excretion of salicylate. *Am. J. vet. Res., 33*:1253–1262.

Dayton, P. G., Cucinell, S. A., Weiss, M., and Perel, J. M. (1967): Dose dependence of drug plasma level decline in dogs. *J. Pharmacol. exp. Ther., 158*:305–316.

Gibaldi, M. (1969): Effect of mode of administration on drug distribution in a two-compartment open system. *J. pharm. Sci., 58*:327–331.

Gibaldi, M., Levy, G., and Weintraub, H. (1971): Drug distribution and pharmacologic effects. *Clin. Pharmacol. Ther., 12*:734–742.

Gibaldi, M., Nagashima, R., and Levy, G. (1969): Relationship between drug concentration in plasma or serum and amount of drug in the body. *J. pharm. Sci., 58*:193–197.

Gibaldi, M., and Perrier, D. (1975): *Pharmacokinetics.* New York, Marcel Dekker.

Gibaldi, M., Schwartz, M. A., and Plaut, M. E. (1968): Serum levels of penicillins: a pharmacokinetic view. *Antimicrob. Agents Chemother.,* pp. 378–381.

Gibaldi, M. and Weintraub, H. (1971): Some considerations as to the determination and significance of biologic half-life. *J. pharm. Sci., 60*:624–626.

Hawkins, R. D., and Kalant, H. (1972): The metabolism of ethanol and its metabolic effects. *Pharmacol. Rev., 24*:67–157.

Jusko, W. J. and Gibaldi, M. (1972): Effects of change in elimination on various parameters of the two-compartment open model. *J. pharm. Sci., 61*:1270–1273.

Kaplan, S. A., Jack, M. L., Alexander, K., and Weinfeld, R. E. (1973): Pharmacokinetic profile of diazepam in man following single intravenous and oral and chronic oral administrations. *J. pharm. Sci., 62*:1789–1796.

Kaplan, S. A., Weinfeld, R. E., Cotler, S., Abruzzo, C. W., and Alexander, K. (1970): Pharmacokinetic profile of trimethoprim in dog and man. *J. pharm. Sci., 59*:358–363.

Kramer, W. G., Lewis, R. P., Cobb, T. C., Forester, W. F., Jr., Visconti, J. A., Wanke, L. A., Boxenbaum, H. G., and Reuning, R. H. (1974): Pharmacokinetics of digoxin: comparison of a two- and a three-compartment model in man. *J. pharmacokinet. Biopharm., 2*:299–312.

Levy, G. (1964): Relationship between elimination rate of drugs and rate of decline of their pharmacologic effects. *J. pharm. Sci., 53*:342–343.

Levy, G. (1965): Pharmacokinetics of salicylate elimination in man. *J. pharm. Sci., 54*:959–967.

Levy, G. (1966): Kinetics of pharmacologic effects. *Clin. Pharmacol. Ther., 7*:362–372.

Levy, G. (1968): Dose dependent effects in pharmacokinetics. *In* D. H. Tedeschi and R. E. Tedeschi (eds.): *Importance of Fundamental Principles in Drug Evaluation.* New York, Raven Press, pp. 141–172.

Levy, G., and Gibaldi, M. (1972): Pharmacokinetics of drug action. *Ann. Rev. Pharmacol., 12*:85–98.

Levy, G., and Nelson, E. (1965): Theoretical relationship between dose, elimination rate and duration of pharmacologic effect of drugs. *J. pharm. Sci., 54*:812

Mercer, H. D., Baggot, J. D., and Sams, R. A. (1977): Application of pharmacokinetic methods to the drug residue profile. *J. Toxicol. env Health 2*:787–801.

Nagashima, R., Levy, G., and O'Reilly, R. A. (1968): Comparative pharmacokinetics of coumarin anticoagulants. *J. pharm. Sci., 57*:1888–1895.

Neff, C. A., Davis, L. E., and Baggot, J. D. (1972): A comparative study of the pharmacokinetics of quinidine. *Am. J. vet. Res., 33*:1521–1525.

Nelson, E. (1961): Kinetics of drug absorption, distribution, metabolism, and excretion. *J. pharm. Sci., 50*:181–192.

Nelson, E., and O'Reilly, I. (1960): Kinetics of sulfisoxazole acetylation and excretion in humans. *J. Pharmacol. exp. Ther., 129*:368–372.

Nielsen, P., and Rasmussen, F. (1972): Elimination of trimethoprim in pigs and goats. *Acta Pharmacol. Toxicol., 31*(Suppl. 1):94.

Notari, R. E. (1973): Pharmacokinetics and molecular modification: implications in drug design and evaluation. *J. pharm. Sci., 62*:865–881.

Pennington, J. E., Dale, D. C., Reynolds, H. Y., and MacLowry, J. D. (1975): Gentamicin sulfate pharmacokinetics: lower levels of gentamicin in blood during fever. *J. inf. Dis., 132*:270–275.

Perrier, D., and Gibaldi, M. (1973): Relationship between plasma or serum drug concentration and amount of drug in the body at steady state upon multiple dosing. *J. pharmacokinet. Biopharm., 1*:17–22.

Piperno. E., Ellis, D. J., Getty, S. M., and Brody, T. M. (1968): Plasma and urine levels of phenylbutazone in the horse. *J. Am. vet. med. Ass., 153*:195–198.

Remmer, H., Neuhaus, G., and Ibe, K. (1961): Die Eliminationsgeschwindigkeit von Glutethimide (Doriden) beim Menschen. *Naunyn-Schmiedeberg's Archs. exp. Path. Pharmak., 242*:90–95.

Riegelman, S., Loo, J. C. K., and Rowland, M. (1968a): Shortcomings in pharmacokinetic analysis by conceiving the body to exhibit properties of a single compartment. *J. pharm. Sci., 57*:117–123.

Riegelman, S., Loo, J., and Rowland, M. (1968b): Concept of a volume of distribution and possible errors in evaluation of this parameter. *J. pharm. Sci., 57*:128–133.

Rowland, M., Benet, L. Z., and Graham, G. G. (1973): Clearance concepts in pharmacokinetics. *J. pharmacokinet. Biopharm., 1*:123–136.

Tschudi, P. (1972): Elimination, Plasmaproteinbindung und Dosierung einiger Sulfonamide. I. Pferd. *Zbl. vet. Med., (A), 19*:851–861.

Tschudi, P. (1973): Elimination, Plasmaproteinbindung und Dosierung einiger Sulfonamide. III. Untersuchungen beim Schwein. *Zbl. vet. Med., (A), 20*:155–165.

Ueda, C. T., Hirschfeld, D. S., Scheinman, M. M., Rowland, M., Williamson, B. J., and Dzindzio, B. S. (1976): Disposition kinetics of quinidine. *Clin. Pharmacol. Ther., 19*:30–36.

Vaughan, D. P., and Beckett, A. H. (1974): An analysis of the intersubject variation in the metabolism of pentazocine. *J. Pharm. Pharmacol., 26*:789–798.

Wagner, J. G. (1968a): Pharmacokinetics. *Ann. Rev. Pharmacol., 8*:67–94.

Wagner, J. G. (1968b): Kinetics of pharmacologic response. I. Proposed relationships between response and drug concentration in the intact animal and man. *J. theoret. Biol., 20*:173–201.

Wagner, J. G. (1973): A modern view of pharmacokinetics. *J. pharmacokinet. Biopharm., 1*:363–401.

Wagner, J. G., Wilkinson, P. K., Sedman, A. J., Kay, D. R., and Weidler, D. J. (1976): Elimination of alcohol from human blood. *J. pharm. Sci., 65*:152–154.

Yeary, R. A., and Swanson, W. (1973): Aspirin dosages for the cat. *J. Am. vet. med. Ass., 163*:1177–1178.

7

Some Important Principles of Drug Dosage

INTRODUCTION

Dose is a quantitative term estimating the amount of drug which must be administered to produce a particular biological response — that is, to establish a certain effective concentration of drug in the body fluids. Factors that influence the concentration attained at the drug's site of action include the dose administered, the route of administration, release and absorption of drug from dosage form (drug product), extent of distribution, penetration to receptors (usually by passive diffusion) and rate of elimination (Fig. 7–1).

Single-dose studies of drug disposition and bioavailability from nonintravascular dosage forms provide quantitative information upon which predictions for multiple dosage regimens can be based. Maintenance of therapeutic amounts of drug in the body requires that the priming and maintenance doses be given at dosage intervals that will keep the amount above a minimum effective level and below a level producing excessive side-effects and toxicity. For therapeutic substances that have a reversible action there exists a range of plasma

190

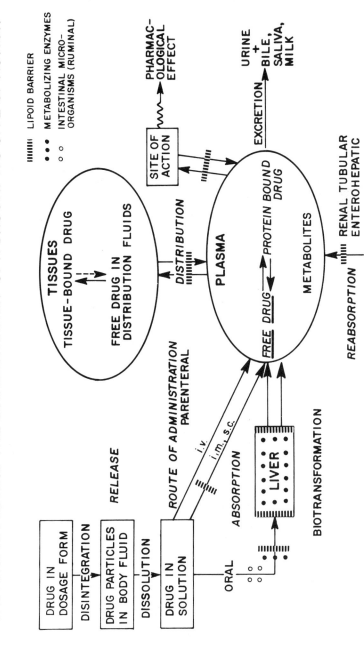

Figure 7–1 Schematic representation of the interrelationship of factors affecting the concentration of a drug at its site of action.

drug concentrations relating to the level in the immediate vicinity of the site of action. This involves the assumption that once pseudo-distribution equilibrium has been attained, changes in the drug concentration in plasma are accompanied by corresponding changes in concentration at the site of action and in the number of drug-receptor interactions. The therapeutic (effective and safe) plasma concentration range, together with the principal pharmacological effect, of a number of drugs is given in Table 7–1. For drugs that exert a pharmacological effect the therapeutic range is obtained by careful clinical evaluation of the response in a sufficient number of appropriately selected individuals, and for antimicrobial agents the range is based upon the minimum inhibitory concentration for susceptible bacteria. Plasma levels of drugs which do not have a rapidly reversible action reveal little about their therapeutic activity (e.g., reserpine). The data in Table 7–1 are derived from the acceptable levels in human therapeutics, since there is a paucity of relevant information on drug dosage in veterinary medicine.

Table 7–1   TENTATIVE RANGES OF THERAPEUTIC PLASMA (OR SERUM) CONCENTRATIONS OF VARIOUS DRUGS

Drug	Usual Range of Therapeutic Plasma Concentrations (μg/ml)	Principal Pharmacological Effect
Salicylate	50–100	Analgesic
	200–350	Antiarthritic
Acetaminophen	10–20	Analgesic
Pentazocine	0.04–0.16	Analgesic
Phenytoin	10–20	Anticonvulsive
Procainamide	4–8	Antiarrhythmic
Lidocaine	1.25–5	Antiarrhythmic
Quinidine	2–5	Antiarrhythmic
Propranolol	0.02–0.08	β-Adrenergic blockade
Digitoxin	0.012–0.030	Sinus stabilizer
Digoxin	0.001–0.003	Rhythm inducer and antiarrhythmic
Antimicrobial Agents*		*Effect*
Sulfonamides	50–150	Bacteriostatic
Trimethoprim	2–6	Bacteriostatic
Chloramphenicol	5–15	Bacteriostatic
Tetracyclines	1.5–4	Bacteriostatic
Erythromycin	2–8	Bacteriostatic
Kanamycin	4–32	Bactericidal
Gentamicin	4–16	Bactericidal
Penicillins	0.1–25	Bactericidal

*The minimum effective serum level of antimicrobial agents depends upon susceptibility of the particular microorganisms.

Species variations in response to many, but not all, drug products can be attributed to differences in their systemic availability, when administered by oral or nonintravascular parenteral routes, and to disposition kinetics rather than to differences in tissue sensitivity. When pharmacological activity is associated with a metabolite, it is essential to quantitate the metabolite levels in plasma so that its rate of elimination can be determined. There can be considerable variation among species in the rate of formation of an active metabolite and in the amount formed. Biotransformation is probably the most important single cause of species variations in response to similar dosage (mg/kg) with lipid-soluble drugs. The response produced by lipophilic drugs is least predictable in cats, for which there is little information on disposition of drugs. When conjugation (particularly glucuronide formation) is an important pathway in the fate of a drug, the potential toxicity may be higher for cats and the duration of action is usually prolonged. Some pharmacodynamic features peculiar to ruminant animals include slow absorption from the reticulorumen and inactivation of some drugs (e.g., chloramphenicol), either by ruminal microorganisms or the reducing environment, diffusion of organic bases from the systemic circulation into ruminal liquor, and highly efficient hepatic biotransformation reactions. The clinician is responsible for the choice of drug product, selection of the route of administration and the amount of drug introduced into the body, but the particular mechanisms in the animal determine the fate and duration of action of the drug. Consequently, an appreciation of the principles of drug dosage based on disposition kinetics of therapeutic agents in domestic animals can only lead to more rational development of drug products for use in animals and an improvement in veterinary therapeutics.

Medication may entail administration of a single dose of drug (e.g., atropine or morphine when used as pre-anesthetic agents, thiopentone when given as the induction or sole anesthetic) or administration of multiple doses at fixed time intervals (e.g., chemotherapy with antimicrobial agents, treatment of congestive heart failure with cardiac glycosides). Titration by therapeutic response is the most reliable method of drug dosage but requires that the pharmacological effect be quantifiable. Induction of anesthesia with pentobarbitone, given by intravenous injection, in the dog is an example of medication "to effect." A therapeutic regimen for furosemide (Lasix) is based on the intensity of diuretic effect produced by an initial trial dose (2.0 mg/kg for dogs and cats; 0.4 mg/kg for horses), which may be adjusted according to the response obtained. Extracellular fluid volume appears to be the most critical factor in determining the diuretic response to this drug (Kelly et al., 1974).

Drugs are potentially toxic chemical agents which, after correct diagnosis and when given only in proper dosage, are likely to produce beneficial effects. For these reasons, the decision as to whether or not to administer a drug should be based upon careful consideration of the objectives of therapy.

Single Doses

In veterinary medicine several drugs are given as single doses. They include atropine (as pre-anesthetic agent), acetylpromazine, succinylcholine, ketamine, fentanyl and droperidol combination, morphine, naloxone, doxapram, apomorphine, pethidine (meperidine), thiabendazole, tetramisole and other anthelmintics.

Assuming that absorption of drug into the bloodstream from the site of administration is first-order, with the rate of absorption proportional to the concentration of drug remaining to be absorbed, the plasma concentration–time profile can be described mathematically by the equation:

$$C_P = -(A' + B')\, e^{-k_{ab}t} + A'e^{-\alpha t} + B'e^{-\beta t} \quad \textbf{Equation 7 • 1}$$

where C_P is the plasma drug concentration at any time t after dosing, k_{ab} is the absorption rate constant, and the exponents α and β are the distribution and elimination rate constants observed after intravenous dosage. The coefficients A' and B' are not the same as A and B (Equation 6·2), since they are influenced by the rate and extent of absorption. Once the extent of absorption (F) has been determined by comparison of the total areas under the plasma level–time curves obtained after oral (or intramuscular) and intravenous administration of equal doses (D) of the drug to the same animals (Equation 2·1), the coefficients A' and B' can be calculated:

Oral or Intramuscular Dosage

$$A' = \frac{k_{ab} \cdot F \cdot D}{V_c\,(\alpha - \beta)} \cdot \frac{\alpha - k_{21}}{k_{ab} - \alpha} \quad \textbf{Equation 7 • 2}$$

$$B' = \frac{k_{ab} \cdot F \cdot D}{V_c\,(\alpha - \beta)} \cdot \frac{k_{21} - \beta}{k_{ab} - \beta} \quad \textbf{Equation 7 • 3}$$

Intravenous Dosage

$$A = \frac{D(\alpha - k_{21})}{V_c\,(\alpha - \beta)}$$

$$B = \frac{D(k_{21} - \beta)}{V_c\,(\alpha - \beta)}$$

The purpose of a dosage calculation is to provide an estimate of the amount of drug which must be administered to produce an effective concentration in the body fluids for a certain period of time. Administration of a just-effective dose gives the threshold concentration of drug in plasma, $C_{P(min)}$, needed to produce a therapeutic effect, and corresponds to a minimum effective amount of drug in the body:

$$A'_{min} = C_{P(min)} \cdot V'_d \qquad \textbf{Equation 7 • 4}$$

where A'_{min} is the just-effective dose per kilogram and V'_d is the apparent specific volume of distribution of the drug. Intravenous dosage or rapid absorption following drug administration by a nonintravascular route and first-order (exponential) elimination are assumed in this discussion of the duration of drug action after administration of single doses. To produce a therapeutic effect, a dose larger than the just-effective dose must be administered. The duration of a therapeutic level of a drug, $t_{C_{P(ther)}}$, depends upon the ratio of administered dose, A_0, to the just-effective dose, A_{min}, and also upon the overall elimination rate constant, β:

$$t_{C_{P(ther)}} = \frac{ln(A_0/A_{min})}{\beta} \qquad \textbf{Equation 7 • 5}$$

Equation 7·5 shows that the duration of a therapeutically effective drug concentration increases as the logarithm of the amount of drug in the body fluids. The application of this relationship is that geometric increases in dose produce only linear increases in duration of action — i.e., persistence of therapeutically effective plasma levels. Administration of twice the just-effective dose gives a duration of action which is equal to the half-life of the drug. To produce an action (therapeutic levels) equivalent to three times the drug's half-life, it would be necessary to administer eight times the amount of the just-effective dose (Fig. 7–2). For a given dose ratio, the smaller the value of β (i.e., the longer the half-life), the longer will be the duration of drug action. The margin of safety (therapeutic index), which dictates the size of the dose ratio, and the half-life of a drug determine the duration of action after administration of a single dose of the drug either by intravenous injection or by a nonintravascular route that provides rapid absorption. When absorption is slower than elimination, the rate of absorption will determine the duration of drug action so long as a sufficient amount is absorbed to give effective levels. This is the situation that exists with satisfactory depot preparations. The half-life of the drug remains the same, irrespective of the dosage form and route of administration, since absorption and distribution processes precede the terminal phase of drug disposition, on which half-life is based.

Some drugs are poorly available systemically either because of incomplete absorption or because of inactivation. Incomplete absorption may be due to slow dissolution of the drug product at the site of

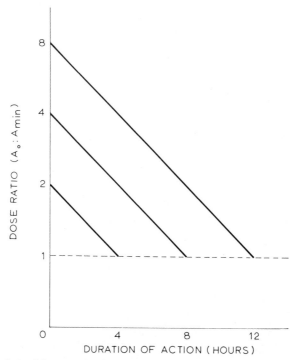

Figure 7–2   Schematic first-order elimination curves for a drug ($t_{1/2} = 4$ hours) depict basis of relationship between dose ratio (ratio of amount of drug administered to just-effective dose) and duration of action. The ordinate could be labeled *plasma drug concentration* (log scale) and the abscissa *time after drug administration* (linear scale). The dashed line would then represent the threshold concentration of drug in plasma required to produce a therapeutic effect rather than the just-effective dose. It is assumed that the duration of action and half-life of the drug coincide.

administration or to physicochemical characteristics of the drug which render it poorly diffusible across a lipoidal membrane. Inactivation may be caused by the acidic reaction in the stomach or be the result of biotransformation by enzymes in the intestinal mucosa and liver (first-pass effect). Dosage requirements are sometimes larger for a drug product given orally than are needed for a parenteral preparation of the same drug.

Dosage Regimen

A systematized dosage schedule is referred to as a dosage regimen. In treating diseases it is usual to administer multiple doses of therapeutic agents (e.g., antipyretics, antimicrobial agents, antihypertensives, antiarrhythmics, anticonvulsants) so that effective drug levels are maintained. A dosage regimen entails two variables: the magnitude of each dose and the frequency with which the dose is repeated, usually expressed as a dosage interval. A regimen which, in theory, should be most effective can be designed for most drug products, provided that a desirable body content of the drug can be clinically defined. The amount of drug in the body which will be effective and safe is determined by the dose-response relationship of the particular compound. The objective in a multiple dosage regimen is to maintain the plasma concentration of the drug within the limits of the maximum safe concentration and the minimum effective level (i.e., within the therapeutic plasma drug concentration range). The effective plasma concentration range of a drug may differ with the indications for therapy (e.g., use of salicylate as an analgesic compared with its use as antiarthritic agent; antimicrobial agents possess activity only against susceptible microorganisms, and minimum effective serum level is variable). The development of a rational dosage regimen for any drug product is governed by the same principles, and is a relatively simple procedure for drugs that have a rapidly reversible action and are eliminated by first-order kinetics. The usual dosage regimen for a drug product assumes that the systemic availability, apparent volume of distribution and half-life of the drug (determined in single dose studies, usually performed in normal animals) are not altered during the course of chronic therapy in diseased animals. Greater consideration should be given to the development of independent dosage regimens for drug products intended for use in each species of domestic animal. Even though the effective concentration range of a drug may be the same in the different species of domestic animals, fractional absorption (systemic availability) from a drug product and values of the disposition parameters may vary widely among the species. Assuming correct diagnosis of a chronic condition, a favorable clinical response is the only real indication of a good choice of therapeutic agent and effectiveness of the dosage regimen.

Therapy with Antimicrobial Agents

Antimicrobial agents behave similarly to other drugs, but their efficacy depends on their ability to act on invading microorganisms rather than on tissue receptors of the host animal. The effective range of levels of an antimicrobial agent in serum is determined by the susceptibility of the invading microorganisms to the particular antibiotic, its degree of penetration (by passive diffusion) to the site of infection, and the margin of safety (ratio of minimum toxic level to effective serum level) of the drug. Ideally, with bacteriostatic agents (sulfonamides, chloramphenicol, tetracycline derivatives, erythromycin), the serum level of free drug (not bound to serum proteins) should not fall below the minimum effective concentration during the course of treatment. The minimum effective concentration of drug in serum (or plasma) is a multiple of the minimum inhibitory concentration (μ) for the particular microorganism, which is determined *in vitro* (Krüger-Thiemer, 1960):

$$C_{P(\text{min})} = \mu \cdot \sigma \qquad \qquad \textbf{Equation 7 • 6}$$

where σ is a safety factor. The value of the safety factor depends upon the class of drug and may be based on the correlation of clinical experience with bacteriological findings — e.g., a safety factor of 10 has been recommended for sulfonamides (Krüger-Thiemer and Bünger, 1965). The success of therapy with bacteriostatic agents depends largely on the activity of the cellular and humoral defense mechanisms of the host. For antibiotics that exert a bactericidal action (penicillins, aminoglycosides), it is unclear whether the area under the serum level–time curve or the peak serum level is the more important. Remission of an infectious disease concurring with antimicrobial therapy is reassuring and suggests that the dosage regimen was completely satisfactory, but this evidence is inconclusive. The optimum conditions for recovery include satisfactory dosage regimen with an antimicrobial agent to which microorganisms are susceptible, reduction of febrile reaction with restoration of normal body temperature, comfortable environment and nursing care.

Steady State Level of Drug

When circumstances necessitate drug therapy, it usually is desirable to rapidly establish an effective concentration of drug in the body and maintain this level for a certain period of time. To achieve this objective, the dosage regimen often consists of an initial priming (or loading) dose, followed by lower maintenance doses, which are administered at fixed time intervals. The priming dose provides an amount of drug in the body that is required to produce an immediate therapeutic effect (Fig. 7–3). Drug levels are maintained within the therapeutic range, $C_{P(\text{ther})} = C_P^\infty{}_{(\text{max})}$ to $C_P^\infty{}_{(\text{min})}$, by administering appropriate maintenance doses at regular intervals thereafter. The dosage interval is normally chosen from among the values of 4, 6, 8, 12 and 24 hours. The same steady state level of a drug can be achieved gradually by ac-

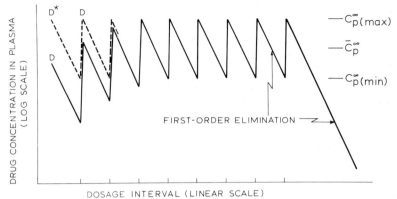

Figure 7–3 A model plot of plasma drug concentration versus time following repeated dosage at fixed intervals of a drug that confers on the body the characteristics of a one-compartment model. Intravenous administration (or other route which provides rapid absorption) and first-order elimination are assumed. Priming dose (D^*) promptly provides a therapeutic level of drug, which can be maintained by administering appropriate maintenance doses at regular intervals. Accumulation of drug by repeated administration of a fixed dose (D) at constant time intervals will eventually achieve the same steady state level. A desirable steady state level may be defined as one within the range of therapeutic plasma drug concentrations. Drug accumulation is a feature of the dosage regimen.

cumulation and without a priming dose. Drug accumulation by repetitive administration of a fixed dose at constant intervals (which are short enough so that complete elimination is not achieved) will eventually produce a therapeutic amount in the body (Boxer et al., 1948; Krüger-Thiemer and Bünger, 1961). When the steady state level has been achieved, each maintenance dose replaces the amount of drug which was eliminated during the preceding interval. Inappropriate choice of either the maintenance dose or the dosage interval will lead to inadequate therapy or to excessive accumulation, with attendant signs of toxicity. With reversibly bound drugs, cumulation is not a property of the drug itself but rather a feature of the dosage regimen. A properly designed and carefully executed multiple dosage regimen ensures effective drug levels throughout the course of treatment and optimizes the probability that therapy will be a success. Dosage regimens based on drug levels require, however, that there exist a well-defined relationship between plasma (or serum) levels of drug and pharmacological or antimicrobial effects (Perrier and Gibaldi, 1974).

Prediction of the average steady state plasma concentration of a drug, under a variety of dosage regimens, may be made by using quantitative information ($t_{1/2}$, V'_d, F) obtained from single dose studies

(Wagner and Metzler, 1969). When a fixed dose of a drug is administered repeatedly at constant time intervals, a steady state will eventually be established in which the plasma level–time curves will be the same during successive dosage intervals (Wagner et al., 1965). Based on this concept one can predict the average steady state amount of drug in the body, $\overline{A}_B^{\infty}$, during a fixed dose–constant interval regimen:

$$\overline{A}_B^{\infty} = \frac{F \cdot D}{\beta \cdot \tau} = \frac{(1.44) \, t_{1/2} \cdot F \cdot D}{\tau} \qquad \textbf{Equation 7 • 7}$$

where $F \cdot D$ is the absorbed dose (F represents the fraction of each dose, D, reaching the systemic circulation intact) and τ is the dosage interval. Calculation of the fractional absorption (F) for nonintravascular routes of administration and the overall elimination rate constant (β) requires a pharmacokinetic study of the drug after intravenous administration. Since $\overline{A}_B^{\infty} = \overline{C}_P^{\infty} \cdot V_{d(area)}$, the average steady state plasma concentration of drug, $\overline{C}_P^{\infty}$, attained during a multiple dosage regimen can be calculated as follows:

$$\overline{C}_P^{\infty} = \frac{F \cdot D}{\beta \cdot V_{d(area)} \cdot \tau}$$

$$= \frac{F \cdot D}{Cl_B \cdot \tau}$$

$$= \frac{(1.44) \, t_{1/2} \cdot F \cdot D}{V_{d(area)} \cdot \tau} \qquad \textbf{Equation 7 • 8}$$

Equations 7·7 and 7·8 hold true for any route of administration and kinetic model, provided that absorption, distribution and elimination can be described by a set of linear differential equations. Steady state plasma drug concentrations are high when the absorbed dose is large, when the interval between successive doses is short and drug elimination is slow (i.e., half-life is long), or when the apparent volume of distribution is small. Average drug concentration maintained during the steady state is a function of maintenance dosage (dose/dosage interval), half-life and apparent volume of distribution of the drug. Whereas the average steady state concentration of drug can be predicted, the plasma concentration fluctuates (oscillates) about the mean during the interval between doses. The more rapidly each dose enters the systemic circulation (influenced by route of administration), the greater will be the extent of fluctuation about the mean steady state plasma concentration. Assuming that absorption is much faster than the rate of elimination, intermittent dosage at intervals equal to the half-life of the drug will attain (by cumulation) a steady state level within 5 per cent of that predicted after the fifth dose. Prediction of average steady state plasma concentration from levels observed after single doses of the drug involves assumptions that the same fraction of each dose of the multiple dose regimen is absorbed as was absorbed after the single dose, and that the volume of distribution and rate constant of elimination are the same for each dose of the multiple dosage regimen as for the single dose (Wagner and Metzler, 1969).

Dosage Predictions Based on Therapeutic Range of Plasma Concentrations

Another approach in designing a multiple dosage regimen is based on the acceptable fluctuation in steady state drug levels during each dosage interval. If one decides to initiate therapy with a single priming (or loading) dose, and thereby produce an immediate therapeutic effect, the magnitude of the dose must be such as to achieve drug concentrations in the body approaching the maximum desirable steady state level. The priming dose per kilogram of body weight, $D^{*'}$, may be calculated from:

$$D^{*'} = A'_{max} = C^{\infty}_{P(max)} \cdot V'_d \qquad \textbf{Equation 7 • 9}$$

where $C^{\infty}_{P(max)}$ is the maximum desirable concentration of drug in plasma at the steady state and V'_d is the apparent specific volume of distribution (in ml/kg), which may be corrected for drug binding to plasma proteins. The apparent volume of distribution is a proportionality constant that relates the plasma concentration of a drug to the amount present in the body. Once established, the therapeutic amount of drug in the body is maintained by repeated administration of a fixed dose at constant intervals. At the steady state, each maintenance dose replaces the amount of drug eliminated during the preceding dosage interval, so that:

$$\begin{aligned} D' &= A'_{max} \cdot f_{el} \\ &= C^{\infty}_{P(max)} \cdot V'_d \cdot f_{el} \end{aligned} \qquad \textbf{Equation 7 • 10}$$

where D' is the maintenance dose per kilogram of body weight, and f_{el} is the fraction eliminated during a dosage interval. The term f_{el} represents the extent of fluctuation in steady state levels of drug that occurs between successive doses, and may be defined by:

$$f_{el} = (1 - e^{-\beta\tau}) \qquad \textbf{Equation 7 • 11}$$

where β is the overall elimination rate constant and τ is the dosage interval. Calculation of maintenance dose may also be based on minimum effective concentration of drug in plasma, $C_{P\,(min)}^{\infty}$, which is present at the end of each dosage interval:

$$D' = C_{P\,(min)}^{\infty} \cdot V'_d \, (e^{+\beta\tau} - 1) \qquad \textbf{Equation 7 • 12}$$

The maintenance dose is the amount of drug which corresponds to the difference between the priming dose and the amount of drug remaining in the body at the end of the dosage interval.

It is evident that the smaller the value of the overall elimination rate constant (i.e., the longer the half-life) of a drug and/or the shorter the dosage interval, the smaller will be the fluctuation and fraction eliminated between successive doses (Table 7–2).

The half-life and margin of safety of a drug are the factors which determine the dosage interval and acceptable fluctuation in steady state levels of the drug. When the maintenance dose is given at intervals equal to the half-life of a drug, 50 per cent fluctuation will be obtained in plasma concentrations of the drug during the steady state. The degree of fluctuation can be reduced without influencing the mean steady state plasma concentration by reducing maintenance dosage, that is, by reducing dose and dosage interval by the same factor. The wider the extent of fluctuation, or range of therapeutic plasma levels, that is acceptable for a drug, the longer the time that may elapse between successive doses. However, linear increases in dosage interval, expressed in multiples of the half-life of a drug, cause geometric increases in the ratio of $C_{P\,(max)}^{\infty}$ to $C_{P\,(min)}^{\infty}$ (Table 7–3).

The relationship between length of dosage interval and acceptable fluctuation in plasma drug levels may be stated in the following way. If the acceptable ratio of $C_{P(max)}^{\infty}$ to $C_{P(min)}^{\infty}$ for a drug at the steady

Table 7–2 RELATIONSHIP BETWEEN HALF-LIFE, LENGTH OF DOSAGE INTERVAL AND EXTENT OF FLUCTUATION IN STEADY STATE LEVEL (ASSUMING INTRAVENOUS ADMINISTRATION OR OTHER ROUTE WITH RAPID ABSORPTION)

$t_{1/2}$ (hours)	β (hour^{-1})	4	6	8	12	24
			Dosage Interval (hours)			
			Extent of Fluctuation (per cent)			
2	0.3465	75	87.5	93.75	98.4	–
4	0.173	50	64.5	75	87.5	98.4
6	0.116	37	50	60	75	93.75
8	0.087	30	40	50	64.5	87.5
12	0.058	20	30	37	50	75
24	0.029	11	16	20	30	50

Table 7–3 RELATIONSHIP BETWEEN LENGTH OF DOSAGE INTERVAL, EXPRESSED IN MULTIPLES OF HALF-LIFE, AND ACCEPTABLE FLUCTUATION IN PLASMA DRUG LEVELS

Dosage Interval $(\epsilon \cdot t_{1/2})$ Values of ϵ	Plasma Drug Level Ratio $C_{P(max)}^{\infty} : C_{P(min)}^{\infty}$	Fluctuation During Dosage Interval (per cent)
1	2	50
2	4	75
3	8	87.5
4	16	93.75
5	32	96.875

state is 2^ϵ, then the dosage interval should be ϵ times the half-life of the drug. Consider a hypothetical drug with a half-life of 6 hours and an effective range of plasma levels between 2 and 8 $\mu g/ml$. Since the ratio of $C_{P(max)}^{\infty} : C_{P(min)}^{\infty}$ at the steady state is 4, the dosage interval should be 12 hours (i.e., $t_{1/2} \times 2$). Using this regimen, 75 per cent fluctuation will exist in plasma steady state concentrations of the drug. Exact prediction of the extent of fluctuation in steady state levels of drug based on single dose studies requires rapid and complete absorption (usually intravenous dosage) and involves the assumptions that the rate constant of absorption, volume of distribution and overall elimination rate constant of the drug are the same after each dose of the multiple dosage regimen as were found following the single dose.

The extent of drug accumulation during repeated dosage depends upon the relative dosage interval, ϵ, where ϵ is a variable that relates dosage interval to half-life of the drug:

$$\epsilon = \frac{\tau}{t_{1/2}}$$

Equation 7 • 13

The lower the value of ϵ chosen by the clinician, the larger will be the fraction of drug remaining at the end of the dosage interval, f_r, and the greater the degree of accumulation. A semilogarithmic graph of fraction remaining at the end of each dosage interval (f_r) versus the relative dosage interval (ϵ) gives a straight line of slope $-\beta$ (Fig. 7–4), which is described by the equation:

$$f_r = (1 - f_{el}) = e^{-\beta\tau}$$

$$= \frac{1}{e^{0.693\,\epsilon}}$$

Equation 7 • 14

$$= \frac{1}{2^\epsilon}$$

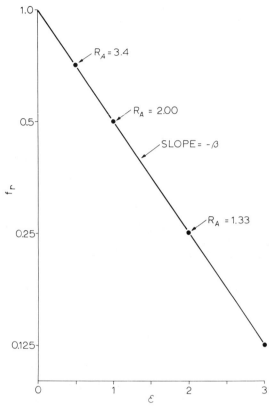

Figure 7–4 A semilogarithmic graph of the fraction remaining at the end of each dosage interval (f_r) versus the relative dosage interval (ϵ) illustrates their relationship. The extent of drug accumulation during repeated dosage becomes greater as the relative dosage interval is reduced. Some values of the accumulation factor (R_A) are shown (see also Table 7–4).

The accumulation factor, R_A, is another useful concept which describes the extent of drug accumulation during a multiple dosage regimen:

$$R_A = \frac{1}{f_{el}} = \frac{1}{(1 - e^{-\beta\tau})} \qquad \textbf{Equation 7 • 15}$$

Some values of the accumulation factor as a function of the relative dosage interval are given in Table 7–4.

When the dosage interval is equal to the half-life ($\epsilon = 1$), the accumulation factor has the value 2.00. When the drug is given in doses at intervals shorter than the half-life ($\epsilon < 1$), the accumulation factor

Table 7-4 THE ACCUMULATION FACTOR AS A FUNCTION OF THE RELATIVE DOSAGE INTERVAL

Accumulation Factor (R_A)	Relative Dosage Interval (ϵ)
145	0.01
14.9	0.1
3.4	0.5
2.00	1.0
1.33	2.0
1.14	3.0
1.07	4.0
1.03	5.0

exceeds 2.00, and when the dosage interval is longer than the half-life ($\epsilon > 1$), the accumulation factor is less than 2.00.

Practical Considerations in Therapeutics

Initiation of therapy with a priming dose and selection of a convenient dosage interval which will enable therapeutic amounts of drug in the body to be maintained are important dosage considerations for drugs with long half-life values (e.g., digitoxin and digoxin), for compounds with a narrow margin of safety (e.g., lidocaine, procainamide, digoxin) and for antimicrobial agents that exert a bacteriostatic effect (e.g., sulfonamides, tetracyclines and chloramphenicol). A practical dosage regimen that would be suitable for most of these drugs (assuming absorption from the drug product to be much faster than the rate of elimination of the drug from the body) is expressed simply in the following relationship:

$$\frac{D^*}{D} = \frac{1}{f_{el}} = \frac{2}{1}$$ **Equation 7 • 16**

This relationship shows that a satisfactory dosage regimen consists of initiating therapy with a priming dose and maintaining therapeutic levels by giving maintenance doses (each half the size of the priming dose) at constant intervals equal to the half-life of the drug. There is no period of inadequate therapy (subtherapeutic levels of drug), and potential toxicity is minimized with this dosage regimen. The dose ratio (D^*/D) is numerically the same as the accumulation factor (R_A). When a priming dose $D^* = R_A \cdot D$ is administered, the steady state level of drug in the body is reached immediately after administration of the first dose.

The pharmacokinetic parameters relevant to dosage of sulfadimethoxine in dogs are given in Table 7–5.

The predicted average steady state concentration of sulfadimethoxine in plasma (Equation 7·8) that would be obtained by administering a fixed dose at constant intervals (24 hours) is presented in Table 7–6.

Using the dosage regimens given in Table 7–6, steady state levels of the drug would not be achieved until after a few days of therapy. The relatively long half-life and bacteriostatic action of sulfadimethoxine indicate that a priming dose should be given to quickly establish a therapeutic amount (20 to 60 mg/kg) of drug in the body. Perhaps the most satisfactory regimen with a 24 hour dosage interval would be to initiate therapy with a priming dose of 55 mg/kg administered by intravenous injection, and maintain therapeutic (safe and bacteriostatic) levels by administering repeatedly, at 24 hour intervals, sulfadimethoxine either intravenously (27.5 mg/kg) or orally (suspension, 55 mg/kg) (Baggot et al., 1976). Maintenance therapy with the oral dosage form would give a lesser degree of fluctuation in steady state levels of sulfadimethoxine. From a theoretical viewpoint, the optimum dosage regimen for sulfadimethoxine would consist of an intravenous priming dose (50 mg/kg) followed by maintenance doses (25 mg/kg) given intravenously at 12 hour dosage intervals. This dosage regimen would be expected to give plasma levels of the drug within the range of 60 to 130 μg/ml throughout the course of therapy.

Administration of a priming dose is unnecessary for drugs with short half-life values (e.g., penicillins and cephalosporins, gentamicin

Table 7–5 PHARMACOKINETICS OF SULFADIMETHOXINE IN BEAGLES ($n=6$) FOLLOWING ADMINISTRATION OF SINGLE DOSES (55 mg/kg) OF SULFADIMETHOXINE BY INTRAVENOUS INJECTION (10 per cent) AND SULFADIMETHOXINE SUSPENSION (12.5 per cent) ORALLY

Kinetic Parameter	Units	Mean $\pm$ S.D.
β	hour^{-1}	0.0538 ± 0.0097
$t_{1/2}$	hours	13.2 ± 2.2
$V'_{d(area)}$	ml/kg	405 ± 63
Cl_B	ml/kg/h	21.4 ± 2.4
$t_{1/2(ab)}$	hours	1.94 ± 0.92
F	per cent	52.4 ± 20.9
$C_{P(12\ hr)}$ (I.V.)	μg/ml	61.5 ± 10.7
$C_{P(24\ hr)}$ (I.V.)	μg/ml	33.0 ± 7.0
$C_{P(12\ hr)}$ (Oral)	μg/ml	36.3 ± 16.2
$C_{P(24\ hr)}$ (Oral)	μg/ml	16.8 ± 8.3
F_b	per cent [100 μg/ml]	80.6 ± 1.1

Table 7-6 TENTATIVE DOSAGE REGIMENS FOR
SULFADIMETHOXINE IN DOGS

Drug Product	Route of Administration	Dose (mg/kg)	Dosage Interval (hours)	$\overline{C}_P^\infty$ (μg/ml)
Sulfadimethoxine	I.V.	55	24	107.5
For Injection	I.V.	27.5	24	53.75
Suspension	Oral	55	24	49.4

and kanamycin). These antibiotics exert a bactericidal effect (i.e., they are irreversibly acting drugs) and the peak serum and tissue levels produced during repetitive dosage may be more critical for these drugs than maintaining levels with bactericidal activity throughout the course of treatment. Apart from differences in bacterial susceptibility, the penicillin analogues and aminoglycoside antibiotics contrast sharply in their margins of safety. Penicillins can be administered in large doses relative to their minimum effective amounts and at wide dosage intervals (up to eight times their half-life values). The half-lives of penicillin G in dogs, cows and horses are 0.5, 0.7 and 0.9 hours, respectively, whereas ampicillin has half-lives of 0.8 hour in dogs, 1.2 hours in cows and 1.5 hours in horses. Multiple dosage regimens with potassium penicillin G or sodium ampicillin, products that are rapidly absorbed from their parenteral sites of administration, usually consist of a series of single doses, since the interval between successive doses is too long to permit accumulation. Gentamicin and kanamycin have relatively narrow ranges of therapeutic (safe and bactericidal) levels in serum which, based on clinical evidence and minimum inhibitory concentrations for susceptible bacteria, may tentatively be set at 4 to 16 μg/ml for gentamicin and 4 to 32 μg/ml for kanamycin. The parenteral dosage forms, which are aqueous solutions of sulfate salts of the bases, are rapidly and completely absorbed from intramuscular sites of administration. The kinetic parameters required for calculation of kanamycin dosage, which were obtained in dogs and horses after parenteral administration of single doses (10 mg/kg) of the drug, are given in Table 7-7.

Based on the data in Table 7-7, usual intramuscular dosage regimens for kanamycin might consist of 10 mg/kg given at 6 hour intervals to dogs and 8 mg/kg every 8 hours for horses. The recommended dosage regimens for kanamycin are a compromise between the need for minimizing the degree of fluctuation to maintain serum levels within therapeutic range and the inconvenience of more frequent dosage. Since the ratio of $C_{P(max)} : C_{P(min)}$ is 2^3, doses would have to

Table 7–7 PHARMACOKINETICS OF KANAMYCIN RELATING TO DOSAGE CALCULATIONS, IN NORMAL DOGS AND HORSES GIVEN SINGLE DOSES (10 mg/kg) OF THE DRUG BY INTRAVENOUS AND INTRAMUSCULAR ROUTES OF INJECTION

Kinetic Parameter	Units	Dog	Horse
β	hour^{-1}	0.7675 ± 0.206	0.4818 ± 0.046
$t_{1/2(\beta)}$	hours	0.970 ± 0.307	1.450 ± 0.148
$V'_{d(area)}$	ml/kg	254.6 ± 30.0	197.9 ± 12.7
Cl_B	ml/kg/min	3.21 ± 0.72	1.59 ± 0.18
$k_{(ab)}$	hour^{-1}	4.6824 ± 0.878	0.6962 ± 0.166
β'	hour^{-1}	0.8234 ± 0.127	0.3517 ± 0.051
F		0.89 ± 0.14	0.95 ± 0.23

be given at intervals of three times $t_{1/2}$ to maintain therapeutic serum levels. The potential toxicity of kanamycin (and other aminoglycosides) limits the size of the dose, so that extension of the dosage interval, as in the recommended regimens, is accompanied by subtherapeutic serum levels for some of the time between successive doses. The half-life and apparent specific volume of distribution of gentamicin in normal dogs are 1.25 hours and 300 ml/kg, respectively, the ratio of $C_{P(max)}:C_{P(min)}$ is 2^2, and F following intramuscular administration is 90 per cent. To establish (by accumulation) and maintain therapeutic serum levels, the theoretical dosage regimen would consist of intramuscular administration of 4 mg/kg every 2.5 hours. A usual clinical dosage regimen might consist of 5 mg/kg given by intramuscular injection at 6 hour intervals. In my opinion, the proposed dosage regimens would be satisfactory in treating infections caused by susceptible microorganisms, and the periods of subtherapeutic levels would not detract significantly from effectiveness of the antibiotics. If a favorable clinical response is not evident after 4 to 5 days of treatment with an aminoglycoside, therapy should be continued with an antibiotic of another class, to which the bacteria were shown to be susceptible. Dosage regimens for treatment of joint infections in the horse, based on pharmacokinetic data and synovial fluid levels of the antibiotics, may consist of intramuscular administration of either gentamicin sulfate (5 mg/kg every 8 hours) or sodium ampicillin (10 mg/kg every 6 hours), depending on susceptibility of infecting bacteria to these antibiotics.

Dosage regimens suitable for chronic therapy with aspirin take into account species differences in rates of absorption and elimination (mainly by metabolism) of salicylate. Appropriate maintenance dosages of aspirin for dogs (25 mg/kg every 8 hours) and cats (25 mg/kg at 24 hour intervals) give serum salicylate levels within the range 100 to 250 μg/ml (Yeary and Swanson, 1973; Yeary and Brant, 1975), which is considered to be a therapeutic range in the human. Even though the systemic availability of salicylate is moderately high (50 to 70 per cent) in cows, the absorption half-time (2.91 hours) is very slow when compared to the half-life (0.54 hour) of the drug. Administration of aspirin to cows at a dosage rate of 100 mg/kg at 12 hour intervals maintained serum salicylate levels of 40 to 60 μg/ml after the third dose (Figs. 7–5 and 7–6). This maintenance dosage was considered (clinical observation) to provide analgesia adequate for relief of mild arthritic conditions in the cows. The dosage interval for aspirin in cows, unlike the interval in regimens for dogs and cats, is based on the rate of absorption rather than on the half-life of salicylate.

Adjustment of Dosage Regimens

Adjustment of the usual dosage regimen is indicated when either the overall elimination rate constant or the apparent volume of distribu-

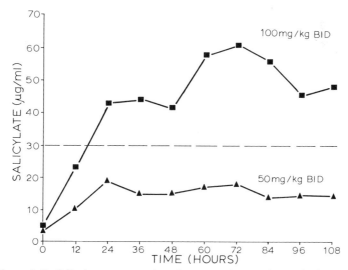

Figure 7–5   Salicylate concentrations in serum of cows after oral administration of aspirin at dosages of 50 mg/kg every 12 hours (▲) and 100 mg/kg every 12 hours (■). Each point is the mean level in three animals. Broken line indicates estimated minimum effective serum salicylate concentration (30 μg/ml). (From Gingerich, D. A., Baggot, J. D., and Yeary, R. A. [1975]: *J. Am. vet. med. Ass., 167*:945–948.)

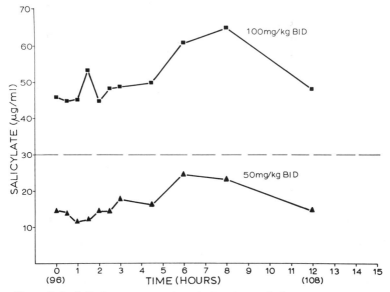

Figure 7–6   Salicylate concentrations during the ninth dosage interval in serum of cows given aspirin orally every 12 hours at the rates of 50 mg/kg (▲) and 100 mg/kg (■). Each point is the mean level in three animals. Broken line indicates estimated minimum effective serum salicylate concentration (30 μg/ml). (From Gingerich, D. A., Baggot, J. D., and Yeary, R. A. [1975]: *J. Am. vet. med. Ass., 167*:945–948.)

tion is significantly altered. It is conceivable that a decrease in one of these kinetic parameters could be compensated for by an increase in the other, so that the net effect on body clearance of the drug would be negligible.

Circumstances which may cause a change in drug disposition include certain types of drug interactions and various disease states. Competitive displacement of extensively (>80 per cent) bound drugs from binding sites on plasma proteins may result in a more intense pharmacological response and usually a shorter duration of action. The activities of the liver microsomal drug-metabolizing enzymes can be markedly increased when animals are treated chronically with any of several drugs (e.g., phenobarbitone, phenylbutazone), steroid hormones, or repeatedly exposed to chlorinated hydrocarbon insecticides. Induction of hepatic microsomal enzymes is important pharmacologically since it causes an accelerated biotransformation of lipid-soluble drugs, and it is of physiological significance because certain endogenous steroids are substrates for the microsomal enzyme systems.

Inhibition of the hepatic microsomal enzyme activity, which is a feature of certain drugs (e.g., quinidine, carbon tetrachloride) and may be a consequence of severe liver disease, would prolong the action of the many therapeutic substances that are eliminated by microsomal oxidation and glucuronide conjugation. Overdosage with organophosphorus compounds, which irreversibly inactivate plasma pseudocholinesterase and inhibit microsomal enzyme systems, causes accumulation of acetylcholine and toxicity. The treatment of poisoning due to cholinesterase inhibition relies upon the principle of blocking the receptors upon which the excessive acetylcholine acts, and the antidote employed for this purpose is atropine. In this situation a considerably larger dose (2 mg/kg) of atropine sulfate should be administered compared with the usual subcutaneous or intramuscular dose (0.04 mg/kg) when given as a pre-anesthetic agent to dogs and cats. Since the phosphoryl-enzyme bond at the esteratic site of cholinesterase is hydrolyzed at a negligible rate, spontaneous recovery is governed by the generation of new enzyme protein, a process which takes several days. To hasten recovery, pralidoxime (50 mg/kg, I.V.; may be repeated after an hour), which is a nucleophilic reactivating agent for phosphorylated cholinesterase, is effective and should be administered in conjunction with atropine. The oxime functions as an antidotal agent by displacing phosphorus from the enzyme (Loomis, 1968).

Particular attention should be given to the selection of a therapeutic agent and to adjustment of the "usual" dosage regimen before initiating therapy in an animal with impaired renal, hepatic or cardiovascular function. Disease states which are known to alter disposition of drugs include uremia, hypoproteinemia, edema and fever. Modification of the dosage regimen involves adjusting maintenance dosage, either by reducing the size of the maintenance dose or increasing the length of the dosage interval. The type of dosage adjustment depends upon the acceptable degree of fluctuation and the mechanism of action of antimicrobial agents. Since the therapeutic amount of drug in the body is independent of the rate of elimination, the priming dose should not be reduced for impaired elimination if the drug is rapidly absorbed, but priming dose must be adjusted for altered volume of distribution. Plasma protein binding of some drugs (e.g., phenytoin, pentobarbitone) is decreased in uremia, and hypoalbuminemia is a feature of hepatic disease. The volume of distribution may be altered during the acute febrile stage of infectious diseases and in animals with congestive heart failure. Whenever a real change in drug distribution occurs, as may be reflected by changes in k_{12}, k_{21}, V_c, and $V_{d(ss)}$, there is cause for concern as to a resulting change in the pharmacological response–plasma concentration relationship. Although a change in $V_{d(B)}$ does not necessarily reflect a real change in distribution, but simply a change in the degree of equilibration of a drug, this change in $V_{d(B)}$ may also, under certain conditions, modify the response–plasma concentration relationship (Gibaldi and Perrier, 1975). In animals with reduced renal function consideration must be given not only to drugs that are excreted mainly unchanged in the urine but also to compounds that are converted to active metabolites which undergo renal excretion.

Elimination of drugs that are excreted predominantly unchanged by the kidneys is slower than normal in animals with impaired renal function. This is reflected by an increase in the half-life values of these drugs (e.g., penicillin G, ampicillin, cephalothin, cephalexin, streptomycin, kanamycin, gentamicin, tobramycin, procainamide, digoxin, furosemide). To avoid the increased risk of toxicity as the consequence of drug accumulation following repeated administration of the usual dose, the dosage regimen has to be modified in accordance with the slower rate of drug elimination (Dettli, 1974; Tozer, 1974; Spring, 1975; Welling et al., 1975). The objective is to reduce the rate of administration to accommodate the slower elimination, so that the same average therapeutic amount of drug in the body is achieved.

Adjustment of dosage regimens for antimicrobial agents may involve lengthening the interval between successive doses (e.g., penicillin G, ampicillin) or reducing the size of the maintenance dose (e.g., sulfonamides, tetracycline, oxytetracycline). It is advisable to make both these adjustments (i.e., reduce size of maintenance dose and increase dosage interval) in dosage regimens for aminoglycoside antibiotics. Since the half-life of aminoglycosides may be considerably increased, it would be beneficial to initiate chemotherapy with a priming dose. It is not necessary to adjust dosage regimens for doxycycline, minocycline, erythromycin, lincomycin, clindamycin and chloramphenicol in animals with impaired renal function, since these antibiotics are eliminated by nonrenal mechanisms.

For drugs with a narrow therapeutic index (e.g., digoxin, procainamide) it is advisable to reduce the size of the maintenance dose and leave dosage interval unchanged, so that a lesser degree of fluctuation in plasma drug levels will be obtained. The priming dose is not altered in the animal with renal impairment, unless there is a real change in volume of distribution, since the same amount of drug is required in the body to produce a therapeutic effect.

Dosage adjustment in renal failure depends upon assessment of the degree of renal impairment (reduction in glomerular filtration rate) which may be estimated by measurement of endogenous creatinine clearance or clearance of ^{125}I-iothalamate (Glofil), obtained by the single injection technique (see *Renal Clearance*, page 120). The constant infusion method for measuring clearance of inulin or ^{125}I-iothalamate is more accurate (Oester et al., 1968) but, in clinical practice, the ease of performing the other methods outweighs the benefit of the more accurate value of GFR. Adjustment of dose is based on the assumption that a linear relationship exists between the overall elimination rate constant of the drug and the endogenous creatinine clearance (Dettli et al., 1971; Perrier and Gibaldi, 1973; Welling, 1975). In patients with renal failure, dosage (even when adjusted) with drugs that have a narrow therapeutic index should be guided by clinical response and monitoring of plasma (or serum) levels on a regular basis.

Unlike renal function, which can be fairly well evaluated by clearance techniques, hepatic drug elimination is not consistently correlated with any of the routine liver function tests. Hepatic drug-metabolizing enzyme activity may be assessed by measurement of the plasma antipyrine half-life (see *Liver Disease and Drug Therapy*, page 102).

Intravenous Infusion

Intravenous infusion is the most desirable mode of administration of drugs that have a narrow range of therapeutic plasma levels (e.g., antiarrhythmic agents, isoproterenol), and it is the only method for maintaining constant (without fluctuation) steady state or plateau levels. When treating a severe infection it might be beneficial to maintain a therapeutic amount of an antibiotic in the body. For antibiotics that are rapidly eliminated (i.e., have short half-lives) maintaining therapeutic levels for a prolonged period of time may require an inconvenient intermittent dosage regimen so that one has to resort to constant rate intravenous infusion. Another aspect of the infusion technique is the latitude which it gives with respect to the intensity of pharmacological response; excessive concentrations, evidenced by appearance of toxic signs, are reduced (by elimination processes) upon stopping the infusion or reducing its rate.

When a drug is given by continuous infusion at a constant rate (zero-order) and disposition (distribution and elimination) within the body is first-order, the level will accumulate until a plateau concentration is reached:

$$C_P = \frac{R_0}{V_c \cdot k_{el}} \left(1 - X_1 e^{-\alpha t} - X_2 e^{-\beta t} \right) \quad \textbf{Equation 7} \bullet \textbf{17}$$

where

$$X_1 = \frac{k_{el} - \beta}{\alpha - \beta}; \ X_2 = \frac{\alpha - k_{el}}{\alpha - \beta}$$

If one assumes the body to behave kinetically as a single homogeneous compartment, then the plasma concentration of drug at any time during infusion is given by:

$$C_P = \frac{R_0}{\beta \cdot V_d} (1 - e^{-\beta t}) \qquad \textbf{Equation 7 • 18}$$

where C_P is the plasma drug concentration at time t, R_0 is the infusion rate (expressed as amount of drug infused per unit time), V_d is the apparent volume of distribution of the drug, and β is the first-order rate constant for overall elimination of drug from the body.

When the plateau level is attained, the steady state plasma drug concentration (C_P^{ss}) is given by the expression:

$$C_P^{ss} = \frac{R_0}{\beta \cdot V_{d(area)}} = \frac{\text{Rate of infusion}}{\text{Body clearance}} \qquad \textbf{Equation 7 • 19}$$

The magnitude of the drug concentration in plasma at the steady state depends on the rate of infusion, the overall elimination rate constant and the apparent volume of distribution of the drug. Since the kinetic constants (β and V_d) are fixed values for a drug, the plateau concentration of drug is directly related to the infusion rate. The time required to reach the plateau concentration depends only upon α and β. For almost all drugs α is considerably larger than β — that is, the half-time of distribution is much shorter than the half-life. Consequently, the rate at which the plateau level is attained during continuous intravenous infusion of a drug at a constant rate depends only upon β or half-life ($t_{1/2} = 0.693/\beta$) of the drug. The time-related approach to a plateau drug level, either from start of an infusion to a given steady state concentration or from a shift (either up or down) from one steady state concentration to another, is given in Table 7–8.

The concentration of drug in the plasma is within 5 per cent of the eventual plateau level after the infusion has continued for a period of five times the half-life of the drug. Doubling the infusion rate leads to a doubling of the plasma concentration at the plateau but does not influence the rate at which the plateau level is attained. Likewise, if the infusion rate is reduced by one-half, the new plateau concentration will be one-half the initial value. The rate at which the drug concentration falls from the initial to the new plateau value is dependent solely upon β, the overall elimination rate constant. In summary, the value of the plateau concentration of a drug in plasma (C_P^{ss}) will be determined by the rate of infusion (R_0), but the rate of approach to the plateau value will always be the same and be determined solely by the overall

Table 7–8 THE RATE OF APPROACH TO PLATEAU
CONCENTRATION DURING CONSTANT INTRAVENOUS
INFUSION OF A DRUG

Duration of Infusion (Multiples of $t_{1/2}$)	Fraction of Plateau Concentration Achieved
1	0.500
2	0.750
3	0.875
4	0.938
5	0.969
6	0.984

elimination rate constant of the drug. When the infusion is terminated, the plasma drug concentration will decline in an exponential fashion, with a half-time for elimination equal to the half-life of the drug.

The rate of infusion which will achieve a desired plateau concentration of drug in the plasma is given by:

$$R'_0 = C_p^{ss} \cdot \beta \cdot V'_{d(ss)} \qquad \textbf{Equation 7 • 20}$$

This equation states that the rate of infusion (μg/min/kg) should be equal to the product of the desired plateau concentration of the drug in plasma and the body clearance value. The plateau plasma drug concentration can be achieved gradually (5 × $t_{1/2}$) by continuous intravenous infusion at a constant rate. When therapeutic considerations require that the plateau concentration be rapidly achieved, either of two techniques may be employed. The classical procedure is to administer a priming dose as an intravenous bolus and, at the same time, start infusing the drug at a constant rate. The priming dose is equal to the infusion rate divided by β:

$$D^* = \frac{R_0}{\beta} \qquad \textbf{Equation 7 • 21}$$

$$= C_p^{ss} \cdot V_{d(ss)}$$

This technique could lead to toxicity with drugs that have a narrow range between toxic and therapeutic plasma levels, as the initial (pre-distribution equilibrium) plasma concentrations may be excessively high. An alternative and safer procedure is to administer the drug by two consecutive constant rate intravenous infusions (Wagner, 1974; Vaughan and Tucker, 1975). An initial constant rate (zero-order) intravenous infusion, at rate R_1, is given over T hours, at which time the rate is abruptly reduced to R_0. The latter infusion rate is then maintained as long as the plateau plasma drug concentration is desired. The final infusion rate (R_0) is calculated by means of Equation 7 · 22. One chooses a time T over which to administer the initial infusion, and then calculates the initial infusion rate (R_1):

$$R_1 = \frac{R_0}{(1 - e^{-\beta T})}$$

Equation 7 • 22

$$\approx \frac{R_0}{\beta T}$$

The duration of initial infusion (T) represents a compromise between immediate attainment of plateau concentration (intravenous bolus) and gradual achievement of desired plateau level by single constant rate infusion. The longer the duration of the initial infusion (0.25 to 3 hours), the lower the ratio of maximum plasma concentration attained at time T to desired plateau plasma drug concentration. This technique requires that drug disposition within the body be described by a linear two-compartment open model, which limits its application to drugs whose plasma concentration–time profiles, after rapid intravenous injection of a single dose, are biexponential. Fortunately, the disposition kinetics of most drugs used in veterinary therapeutics can be satisfactorily described by the two-compartment open model.

Special Dosage Forms

If the maintenance dosage (D/τ) of a drug is impractical, owing to short half-life and narrow range of therapeutic levels, or likely to produce toxic effects when dose is increased to make dosage interval convenient, the drug should be administered either by intravenous infusion or by a special dosage form. Both sustained-release dosage forms and prolonged-action preparations of drugs that have short half-lives provide an extended response (i.e., a longer duration of action) and obviate the need for dosing at short intervals, for administering unduly large doses of the usual drug products or for resorting to an intravenous infusion. Since the amount of drug administered at one time in a unit dose of a special dosage form always exceeds the single dose of the usual product, drugs with narrow therapeutic indices should be administered by intravenous infusion. The potential toxicity of sustained-release preparations of these drugs would be great, since release from dosage form and absorption are unpredictable. Criteria supporting usefulness of a special dosage form should include *in vivo* data showing duration of therapeutic levels of the drug following administration of the recommended dose to the particular species of animal. Assuming the drug is clinically effective, the relative velocities of two rate processes, namely dissolution of the dosage form at site of administration and elimination of the drug from the body, largely determine duration of drug action and response to therapy with a special dosage form. As well as reducing the frequency of dosage, the aim in using these drug preparations is to minimize fluctuations in levels of drug in blood and tissues so that a more uniform pharmacological effect is expected.

Sustained-release dosage forms, in theory, provide an initial therapeutic dose that is available upon administration of the product followed by a gradual release of drug over a prolonged period of time. Variability in drug absorption is a feature of sustained-release dosage forms (Crosland-Taylor et al., 1965). Prolonged-action preparations release the drug at a rate that will provide a significantly longer duration of action than a single dose of the usual product. The (serum) half-life of penicillin G in the cow is 0.7 hour (Ziv et al., 1973). A dose (6 million units, injected intramuscularly) of procaine penicillin G in aqueous solution was shown to provide a serum penicillin level above 0.05 unit/ml for at least 24 hours in the cow (Schipper et al., 1971). Dissolution rather than absorption is the rate-limiting step that determines entry of drugs into the systemic circulation from prolonged-release dosage forms, whether they are intended for oral or parenteral administration. If a uniform rate of release of drug from these preparations is possible, analogous to a constant intravenous infusion, plateau concentrations of drug can be achieved in blood and other tissues. Disadvantages of prolonged-release dosage forms include the loss of flexibility in drug dosage and wide variations in the intensity and duration of drug action.

REFERENCES

Baggot, J. D., Ludden, T. M., and Powers, T. E. (1976): The bioavailability, disposition kinetics and dosage of sulphadimethoxine in dogs. *Can. J. comp. Med.*, *40*:310–317.

Boxer, G. E., Jelinek, V. C., Tompsett, R., DuBois, R., and Edison, A. O. (1948): Streptomycin in the blood: chemical determination after single and repeated intramuscular injections. *J. Pharmacol. exp. Ther.*, *92*:226–235.

Crosland-Taylor, P., Keeling, D. H., and Cromie, B. W. (1965): A trial of slow-release tablets of ferrous sulfate. *Curr. Ther. Res.*, *7*:244–248.

Dettli, L. C. (1974): Drug dosage in patients with renal disease. *Clin. Pharmacol. Ther.*, *16*:274–280.

Dettli, L., Spring, P., and Ryter, S. (1971): Multiple dose kinetics and drug dosage in patients with kidney disease. *Acta Pharmacol. Toxicol.*, *29*(Suppl. 3):211–224.

Gibaldi, M., and Perrier, D. (1975): *Pharmacokinetics.* New York, Marcel Dekker.

Gingerich, D. A., Baggot, J. D., and Yeary, R. A. (1975): Pharmacokinetics and dosage of aspirin in cattle. *J. Am. vet. med. Ass.*, *167*:945–948.

Kelly, M. R., Cutler, R. E., Forrey, A. W., and Kimpel, B. M. (1974): Pharmaco-kinetics of orally administered furosemide. *Clin. Pharmacol. Ther., 15*:178–186.

Krüger-Thiemer, E. (1960): Dosage schedule and pharmacokinetics in chemotherapy. *J. Am. pharm. Assoc., 49*:311–313.

Krüger-Thiemer, E., and Bünger, P. (1961): Kumulation und toxizitat bei falscher dosierung von sulfanilamiden. *Arzneim.-Forsch., 11*:867–874.

Krüger-Thiemer, E., and Bünger, P. (1965): The role of the therapeutic regimen in dosage design. *Chemotherapia, 10*:61–73.

Loomis, T. A. (1968): *Essentials of Toxicology.* Philadelphia, Lea and Febiger.

Oester, A., Olesen, S., and Madsen, P. O. (1968): Determination of glomerular filtration rate: old and new methods. *Invest. Urology, 6*:315–321.

Perrier, D., and Gibaldi, M. (1973): Estimation of drug elimination in renal failure. *J. clin. Pharmacol., 13*:458–462.

Perrier, D., and Gibaldi, M. (1974): Drug concentrations in the plasma as an index of pharmacologic effect. *J. clin. Pharmacol., 14*:415–417.

Schipper, I. A., Filipovs, D., Ebeltoft, H., and Schermeister, L. J. (1971): Blood serum concentrations of various benzyl penicillins after their intramuscular administration to cattle. *J. Am. vet. med. Ass., 158*:494–500.

Spring, P. (1975): Calculation of drug dosage regimens in patients with renal disease: A new nomographic method. *Int. J. clin. Pharmac., 11*:76–80.

Tozer, T. N. (1974): Nomogram for modification of dosage regimens in patients with chronic renal function impairment. *J. pharmacokinet. Biopharm., 2*:13–28.

Vaughan, D. P., and Tucker, G. T. (1975): General theory for rapidly establishing steady state drug concentrations using two consecutive constant rate intravenous infusions. *Europ. J. clin. Pharmac., 9*:235–238.

Wagner, J. G. (1974): A safe method for rapidly achieving plasma concentration plateaus. *Clin. Pharmacol. Ther., 16*:691–700.

Wagner, J. G., and Metzler, C. M. (1969): Prediction of blood levels after multiple doses from single dose blood level data: data generated with two-compartment open model analyzed according to the one-compartment open model. *J. pharm. Sci., 58*:87–92.

Wagner, J. G., Northam, J. I., Alway, C. D., and Carpenter, O. S. (1965): Blood levels of drug at the equilibrium state after multiple dosing. *Nature* (Lond.), *207*:1301–1302.

Welling, P. G. (1975): Dose adjustment in renal failure. *J. pharm. Sci., 64*:175–176.

Welling, P. G., Craig, W. A., and Kunin, C. M. (1975): Prediction of drug dosage in patients with renal failure using data derived from normal subjects. *Clin. Pharmacol. Ther., 18*:45–52.

Yeary, R. A., and Brant, R. J. (1975): Aspirin dosages for the dog. *J. Am. vet. med. Ass., 167*:63–64.

Yeary, R. A., and Swanson, W. (1973): Aspirin dosages for the cat. *J. Am. vet. med. Ass., 163*:1177–1178.

Ziv, G., Shani, J., and Sulman, F. G. (1973): Pharmacokinetic evaluation of penicillin and cephalosporin derivatives in serum and milk of lactating cows and ewes. *Am. J. vet. Res., 34*:1561–1565.

8

Drug Therapy in the Neonatal Animal

INTRODUCTION

It is well known that the newborn and young of mammalian species are more sensitive or susceptible to the toxic effects of various drugs than are adults (Done, 1964). Central nervous system depressants such as chloral hydrate, phenobarbital, meprobamate and chlorpromazine appear to be more toxic to the neonate than to the adult. Morphine is considerably more toxic in the neonate, whereas meperidine has about the same LD_{50} in both newborn and mature animals. Specific receptors in the brain may be more sensitive to morphine in the immature animal (Mirkin, 1970). Certain stimulants of the central nervous system (strychnine, d-amphetamine and pentylenetetrazol) have a significantly lower LD_{50} in the neonatal than in the adult rat (Yeary, 1967). Many, if not most, of the aberrant responses shown by the immature animal to foreign organic compounds can undoubtedly be attributed to differences in drug disposition. Alteration in the pattern of distribution may be related to the relative volumes of the fluid compartments of the body. Neonatal hypoalbuminemia causes low extent of binding to plasma albumin and leaves a larger fraction of the dose available for distribution. The blood-brain

219

barrier is underdeveloped at birth in many animal species (Davson, 1967), so that compounds with restricted access to the brain of the adult will permeate tissues of the central nervous system of the neonatal animal. Marked deficiencies in the processes of elimination (metabolic and excretory) and rapid development of enzyme systems are characteristic features of the neonatal period. This period may be defined as the time span from birth to one month of age.

BIOTRANSFORMATION

In the newborn, certain drug-metabolizing enzymes take a few weeks to develop (Brown et al., 1958). Biotransformation pathways associated with the microsomal drug-metabolizing enzyme systems (i.e., oxidation and reduction reactions and glucuronic acid conjugation) are deficient in infants and neonatal animals. The postnatal pattern of development of drug-metabolizing enzymes in the liver appears to be biphasic in nature, consisting of a rapid and nearly linear increase in activity during the first three to four weeks, which is followed by slower development up to the tenth week postpartum. The carbon monoxide–binding pigment, cytochrome P-450, of hepatic microsomes was shown to develop in parallel with the oxidative and reductive pathways, suggesting that this cytochrome may be rate-limiting to the development of these biotransformation pathways (Short and Davis, 1970). It is conceivable that the pattern of development of microsomal enzyme systems during the neonatal period is similar among all mammalian species. Both steroid (hydrocortisone) and polypeptide (growth) hormones may affect the normal postnatal development of hepatic microsomal enzyme activity (Wilson, 1972; Mukhtar et al., 1974). The ability to synthesize glucuronide conjugates develops rapidly during the neonatal period. The levels of glucuronyl transferases (microsomal enzyme) in the newborn of most species, with the exception of the rat, are remarkably low (Dutton, 1966). Formation of the "activated" nucleotide uridine diphosphate glucuronic acid (UDPGA) from uridine diphosphate glucose is catalyzed by UDPG-dehydrogenase, an enzyme found in the supernatant fraction of liver preparations (Dutton, 1961). This enzyme has low activity in newborn animals (Grodsky et al., 1958; Dutton, 1959; Arias et al., 1963). Consequently, defective glucuronide synthesis in the newborn is due to low activity of the enzyme that catalyzes formation of the "activated" nucleotide (UDPGA) and deficiency of microsomal glucuronyl transferase. Unlike its relative inability to form glucuronide conjugates, the neonate apparently possesses acetylation capabilities like those of the normal adult (Vest and Rossier, 1963).

PLASMA PROTEIN BINDING

Large differences between adult and neonatal plasma albumin concentrations could be expected to produce appreciable age-related variations in the amount of free drug in the circulation and in the fraction available for distribution. Salicylic acid is very poorly bound to proteins of fetal plasma; the percentage of drug bound increases markedly during the first week postpartum, and is followed by a further increase between the first and fourth weeks (Short and Tumbleson, 1973). The binding pattern of salicylate parallels the rise in albumin concentration of plasma that occurs during the neonatal period. The binding of pentobarbital and thiopental presented a different developmental profile from that of salicylate and does not appear to be a function of albumin concentration alone. The barbiturate concentration–dependent spread in binding values decreased markedly to attain a pattern similar to that of the adult by the first week postpartum. Binding studies of various drugs to human adult and placental cord plasma have shown a relative hypoalbuminemia and concomitant decrease in the fraction of drug bound to placental cord plasma proteins (Ehrnebo et al., 1971; Chignell et al., 1971; Pruitt and Dayton, 1971).

EXCRETION

Renal function, as determined by clearances of inulin and para-aminohippuric acid (which are indicative of glomerular filtration rate and effective renal plasma flow, respectively), is relatively inefficient in neonatal animals of most species, including humans. The elimination half-time for inulin is about three times longer in the infant compared with the human adult, suggesting some partial impermeability of the glomerular membrane or, more likely, a smaller renal blood flow relative to the body water volume. More striking is the deficiency in PAH excretion (tubular secretion); the elimination half-time of this compound is nearly four times longer in the infant than in the adult (Goldstein et al., 1974). It is important to appreciate, however, that whereas neonatal renal capacity may be "immature" relative to that of the adult, it is, nevertheless, adequate for the functions it normally has to perform. The delayed elimination of N-acetyl-p-aminophenol (acetaminophen) by newborn infants has been shown to be caused not only by retarded conjugation with glucuronic acid, but also by diminished urinary excretion of the conjugate (Mereu et al., 1962; Vest and Rossier, 1963).

The neonatal calf, unlike most other newborn animals and human infants, has an efficient renal function with respect to the production of concentrated urine, excretion of excess fluid and urea clearance (Dalton, 1966, 1967, 1968a,b). Moreover, clearance values (mean $\pm$ S.D., $n = 15$) of inulin (130 $\pm$ 26 ml/min/1.73 m^2) and p-aminohippurate (592 $\pm$ 177 ml/min/1.73 m^2), which measure glomerular filtration rate and renal plasma flow, respectively, obtained in calves aged 2 to 20 days are comparable to those of human adults. Values in the calf were considered to be also comparable to those in the adult cow when due allowance was made for the bias introduced when comparing subjects so greatly different in size (Dalton, 1968c).

There is evidence that there may be a hepatic excretory defect in the newborn, at least in regard to bilirubin (Schenker, 1963; Schenker and Schmid, 1964; Schenker et al., 1964) and Bromsulphalein (Sussmann et al., 1962; Vest and Rossier, 1963). This defect may tentatively be attributed to a combination of retarded conjugation reactions in hepatic cells and inefficient carrier-mediated transfer processes for transport of substances into bile. Whatever the mechanisms, it is apparent that the elimination of many drugs from the body is delayed in the neonate as major pathways of biotransformation operate at a reduced rate and excretion processes (particularly carrier-mediated transport) are inefficient.

DRUG THERAPY

Drug therapy in the neonate deserves special consideration and should be initiated only when the life of the animal is endangered. Computation of the size of the dose to be administered must take into account the desired plasma level and extent of distribution in the neonatal animal. The reduced degree of binding to plasma proteins, the relative volumes of the body fluid compartments and permeability of the blood-brain barrier influence the distribution of the drug and sensitivity of the animal to the effects. Although the size of the initial dose determines the amount of drug in the body at the commencement of therapy, the frequency of dosage will determine the degree of drug accumulation and potential toxicity. Since drug elimination is delayed, the interval between successive doses must be extended. Owing to probable immunodeficiency in the neonate, use of antimicrobial agents that have a bactericidal action would be preferred for treatment of bacterial infections. Because of the increased risk associated with drug therapy during the neonatal period, the selection of an antimicrobial agent should be based on susceptibility of infecting microorganisms, mechanism of action and fate (mechanisms of elimination) of the drug, and the therapeutic index. The penicillin analogues, in particular ampicillin, should be the first class of antimicrobial agents considered. The extent of absorption of ampicillin from oral dosage forms may be considerably greater during the neonatal period. In neonates of all species except the calf, ampicillin may be dosed at 24 hour intervals. In calves, a dosage interval of 8 or 12 hours should be employed. Because of their relatively narrow margin of safety, use of aminoglycoside antibiotics should generally be avoided in the newborn. When, however, the infecting microorganisms are particularly susceptible to aminoglycosides, kanamycin or gentamicin may be administered, parenterally for systemic infections, at 24 hour intervals.

The inability to diurese and the low renal clearance can become critical factors when administering fluid and electrolytes therapeutically. It is generally advisable to avoid giving isotonic saline solution. One should administer *per os* a hypotonic electrolyte solution ($\frac{1}{4}$ to $\frac{1}{2}$ dilution of physiological saline solution) containing 5 to 10 per cent glucose. This should be given in small repeated doses. The volume of fluid administered depends on the clinical condition of the animal, but generally the total fluid intake per day should be equivalent to 10 to 15 per cent of the body weight.

REFERENCES

Arias, I. M., Gartner, L., Furman, M., and Wolfson, S. (1963): Studies of the effect of several drugs on hepatic glucuronide formation in newborn rats and humans. *Ann. N.Y. Acad. Sci., 111*:274–279.
Brown, A. K., Zuelzer, W. W., and Burnett, H. H. (1958): Studies with neonatal development of the glucuronide conjugating system. *J. clin. Invest., 37*:332–340.
Chignell, C. P., Vesell, E. S., Starkweather, D. K., and Berlin, C. M. (1971): The binding of sulfaphenazole to fetal, neonatal, and adult human plasma albumin. *Clin. Pharmacol. Ther., 12*:897–901.
Dalton, R. G. (1966): Production of hypertonic urine by the calf. *Vet. Rec., 79*:53–54.
Dalton, R. G. (1967): The effect of starvation on the fluid and electrolyte metabolism of neonatal calves. *Brit. vet. J., 123*:237–246.
Dalton, R. G. (1968a): Renal function in neonatal calves: diuresis. *Brit. vet. J., 124*:371–381.
Dalton, R. G. (1968b): Renal function in neonatal calves: urea clearance. *Brit. vet. J., 124*:451–459.
Dalton, R. G. (1968c): Renal function in neonatal calves: inulin, thiosulphate and para-aminohippuric acid clearance. *Brit. vet. J., 124*:498–502.
Davson, H. (1967): *Physiology of the Cerebrospinal Fluid.* London, Churchill.
Done, A. K. (1964): Developmental pharmacology. *Clin. Pharmacol. Ther., 5*:432–479.
Dutton, G. J. (1959): Glucuronide synthesis in foetal liver and other tissues. *Biochem. J., 71*:141–148.
Dutton, G. J. (1961): The mechanism of glucuronide formation. *Biochem. Pharmacol., 6*:65–71.
Dutton, G. J. (1966): The biosynthesis of glucuronides. *In* G. J. Dutton (ed.): *Glucuronic Acid, Free and Combined. Chemistry, Biochemistry, Pharmacology and Medicine.* Academic Press, New York, pp. 185–299.

Ehrnebo, M., Agurell, S., Jalling, B., and Boréus, L. O. (1971): Age differences in drug binding plasma proteins: Studies on human fetuses, neonates and adults. *Europ. J. clin. Pharmacol., 3*:189–193.

Goldstein, A., Aronow, L., and Kalman, S. M. (1974): *Principles of Drug Action: The Basis of Pharmacology.* 2nd Ed. New York, John Wiley & Sons.

Grodsky, G. M., Carbone, J. V., and Fanska, R. (1958): Enzymatic defect in metabolism of bilirubin in foetal and newborn rat. *Proc. Soc. exp. Biol. Med., 97*:291–294.

Mereu, T., Apollonio, T., Sereni-Piceni, L., and Careddu, P. (1962): Research on the urinary elimination of N-acetyl-*p*-aminophenol (NAPA) in newborn infants. II. Renal factors influencing the elimination of free NAPA and its conjugates. *Minerva Pediat., 14*:1047–1049.

Mirkin, B. L. (1970): Developmental pharmacology. *Ann. Rev. Pharmacol., 10*:255–272.

Mukhtar, H., Sahib, M. K., and Kidwai, J. R. (1974): Precocious induction of hepatic aniline hydroxylase and aminopyrine N-demethylase with hydrocortisone in neonatal rat. *Biochem. Pharmacol., 23*:345–349.

Pruitt, A. W., and Dayton, P. F. (1971): A comparison of the binding of drugs to adult and cord plasma. *Europ. J. clin. Pharmacol., 4*:59–62.

Schenker, S. (1963): Disposition of bilirubin in the fetus and the newborn. *Ann. N.Y. Acad. Sci., 111*:303–305.

Schenker, S., and Schmid, R. (1964): Excretion of ^{14}C-bilirubin in newborn guinea pigs. *Proc. Soc. exp. Biol. Med., 115*:446–448.

Schenker, S., Daber, N. H., and Schmid, R. (1964): Bilirubin metabolism in the fetus. *J. clin. Invest., 43*:32–39.

Short, C. R., and Davis, L. E. (1970): Perinatal development of drug-metabolizing enzyme activity in swine. *J. Pharmacol. exp. Ther., 174*:185–196.

Short, C. R., and Tumbleson, M. E. (1973): Binding of drugs to plasma proteins of swine during the perinatal period. *Toxicol. appl. Pharmacol., 24*:612–624.

Sussman, S., Carbone, J. V., Grodsky, G., Hjelte, V., and Miller, P. (1962): Sulfobromophthalein sodium metabolism in newborn infants. *Pediatrics, 29*:899–906.

Vest, M. F., and Rossier, R. (1963): Detoxification in the newborn: the ability of the newborn infant to form conjugates with glucuronic acid, glycine, acetate and glutathione. *Ann. N.Y. Acad. Sci., 111*:183–197.

Wilson, J. T. (1972): Developmental pharmacology: a review of its application to clinical and basic science. *Ann. Rev. Pharmacol., 12*:423–450.

Yeary, R. A. (1967): Drug toxicity in newborn animals. *Appl. Ther., 9*:918–921.

GLOSSARY

Pharmacokinetic analysis of drug concentration in plasma versus time data after administration of an intravenous bolus dose yields the hybrid parameters P, A, B (coefficients) and π, α, β (rate constants) directly, and the microconstants (k_{12}, k_{21}, k_{13}, k_{31}, k_{el}) associated with a multicompartment open model by calculation. Coefficients are in units of concentration (μg/ml) and rate constants are expressed in units of reciprocal time (min^{-1} or hour^{-1}).

A_0 — Amount of drug in the body (central compartment) immediately following intravenous injection of a single dose; dose administered.

A_{min}	Just-effective dose; minimum effective amount of drug in the body.
$\bar{A}_B^{\infty}$	Average amount of drug in the body at steady state during a multiple dose regimen.
A_B^{ss}	Amount of drug in the body at infusion equilibrium (plateau level) during constant rate (zero-order) intravenous infusion.
$A_{B(t)}$	Amount of drug in the body at time t.
A_c, A_T	Amount of drug in the central and peripheral (tissue) compartments at time t.
A, B	Zero-time plasma drug concentration intercepts of biphasic intravenous disposition curve. The coefficient B is based on the terminal exponential phase.
α, β	Hybrid rate constants of biphasic intravenous disposition curve. Values of α and β are related to the slopes of distribution and elimination phases, respectively, of biexponential drug disposition curve. Beta (β) is the overall elimination rate constant and is obtained from the terminal slope of a semilogarithmic plot of plasma drug concentration versus time; the expression $0.693/\beta$ is the (biological) half-life of a drug that undergoes exponential (first-order) elimination.
β^1	Apparent overall elimination rate constant obtained from terminal slope of a semilogarithmic plot following drug administration by a nonintravascular route.
Area, AUC, $\int_0^{\infty} C_P\, dt$	Total area under the plasma drug concentration versus time curve from $t=0$ to $t=\infty$ after administration of a single dose.
$\int_0^t C_P\, dt$	Area under the plasma drug concentration versus time curve from time zero to t.
C_P^0	Plasma drug concentration immediately following intravenous injection of a single dose. Initial concentration of drug in plasma following administration of an intravenous bolus dose.
C_P	Drug concentration in the plasma at time t.
C_T	Drug concentration in distribution fluids (tissues) at time t.
C_P^{ss}	Plateau (steady state) concentration of drug

	in the plasma during constant rate (zero-order) intravenous infusion.
$C_{P(max)}^{\infty}, \; \overline{C}_P^{\infty}, \; C_{P(min)}^{\infty}$	Maximum desirable, average and minimum effective concentrations of drug in the plasma at steady state during a multiple dose regimen.
$C_{P(ther)}$	Therapeutic range of plasma drug concentrations.
$C_{P(t*)}$	Last measured concentration of drug in the plasma following administration of a single dose.
Cl_B	Body clearance of a drug, which represents the sum of all clearance processes in the body.
D	Maintenance dose.
$D*$	Priming (or loading) dose.
D/τ	Maintenance dosage.
dC_P/dt	Rate of change of drug concentration in the plasma.
dA_B/dt	Rate of change of drug level in the body.
e	Base of natural logarithm (ln).
ϵ	Relative dosage interval.
F	Fraction of administered dose which reaches the systemic (general) circulation intact (i.e., fraction available systemically). In some cases, F may represent extent of drug absorption.
F_b	Fraction of drug bound to plasma (or serum) proteins.
f_c	Fraction of drug in the body that is contained in the central compartment.
f_{el}	Fraction eliminated during a dosage interval. This term represents the extent of fluctuation in steady state levels of drug that takes place between successive doses.
f_r	Fraction remaining at the end of a dosage interval.
K_a	Equilibrium association constant of drug-albumin interaction.
K_d	Dissociation constant of drug-albumin complex.
K_m	Michaelis constant.
k_{ab}	Apparent first-order absorption rate constant.

k_{el}	First-order elimination rate constant for disappearance of drug from the central compartment.
k_{12}, k_{21}, k_{13}, k_{31}	First-order transfer rate constants for drug distribution between the central and peripheral compartments.
n	Number of animals used in a drug disposition study; number of binding sites on plasma albumin.
pK_a	Negative logarithm of (acid) dissociation constant of an organic electrolyte (used for both acids and bases).
R_A	Accumulation factor describing extent of drug accumulation in a multiple dosage regimen.
R_0, R_1	Constant rate (zero-order) intravenous infusion; infusion rate.
$R_{x/y}$	Theoretical equilibrium concentration ratio of a drug on opposite sides (x and y) of a biological membrane.
r	Moles of drug bound per mole of albumin.
$[S]$	Substrate concentration.
τ	Dosage interval.
t	Time.
t_d	Duration of a pharmacological effect.
$t_{C_{P(\text{ther})}}$	Duration of therapeutic plasma level of a drug.
t^*	Time at which the last blood sample was collected.
T	Duration of a constant rate intravenous infusion (from 0 to T hours); T denotes time at which infusion is terminated.
$t_{1/2(ab)}$	Absorption half-time ($0.693/k_{ab}$).
$t_{1/2(\alpha)}$	Distribution half-time.
$t_{1/2(\beta)} = t_{1/2}$	Elimination half-time. This term is the (biological, plasma) half-life of a drug ($0.693/\beta$).
v	Velocity of an enzyme-catalyzed reaction.
V_{max}	Maximum velocity of process described by Michaelis-Menten kinetics.
V_c	Apparent volume of the central compartment.
V_d	Apparent volume of distribution of a drug (liters); proportionality constant relating the plasma concentration of a drug to the amount of drug in the body.

V_d'	Apparent specific volume of distribution of a drug (liters/kg).
$V_{d(B)}$	Apparent volume of drug distribution obtained by neglecting the α (distributive) phase of drug disposition (extrapolation method).
$V_{d(\text{area})}$	Apparent volume of drug distribution based on total area under the plasma drug concentration versus time curve (area method).
$V_{d(ss)}$	Steady state volume of distribution of a drug. Can be used to estimate amount of drug in the body at infusion equilibrium (plateau) and during steady state upon repetitive dosing.

Index

Page numbers in *italics* refer to illustrations; (t) indicates tables.

229